Making a Good L

What does it mean to be a good doctor? How do we learn to respond well to suffering—both our patients' and our own—and to sustain ourselves in systems that so often undermine those very values we must hold on to?

In this anthology a group of physicians from five countries—ranging from newly qualified doctors to internationally recognized scholars—come together to reflect on the tensions and promises of current medical education and practice. *Making a Good Doctor* is a weave of academic inquiry, personal narrative, literary reflection, and pedagogical dialogue.

Across eighteen chapters, the book explores the emergence of medicalization, over-diagnosis, alienation, burnout, moral injury, and the commodification of care. It celebrates the joy of medicine, its power to heal—the transformative force of listening, of dialogue, of shared presence.

Key Features

- Offers a uniquely holistic combination of personal stories and critical perspectives on current medical education and practice
- Builds around a person-centred ideal that sets the humanity of both patients and professionals at the centre of medical education and practice
- Expresses ideas and ideals that have been tested in educational practice and have solid theoretical underpinnings in medical philosophy and psychological and pedagogical research

This book is directed toward the medical practitioner, educator, or student interested in understanding more about the forces that shape, and distort, medical culture and healthcare systems. It is for those interested in developing insight; in learning techniques for collaboration, resistance, resilience, and change.

This is an absolutely uplifting book.

Doctors will love this book. It speaks to them in profoundly personal ways, and also in stimulating intellectual ways. It contains affirming messages from 14 doctors of all ages from 5 countries, written in a creative array of formats, poems, dialogues, email exchanges, [and] formal chapters. Also, some writings are full of source material to help doctors and educators shape a better world in medicine. You, the reader, will feel deeply heard as everyday issues are addressed head on—a perfect antidote to discouragement and burnout. You no longer feel alone as you are invited to immerse yourself in the tough stuff when the authors share their distress. Through honesty, they come to a place of wisdom and hope.

Moira Stewart, PhD
Distinguished University Professor Emeritus
Centre for Studies in Family Medicine
Western University
Canada

Making a Good Doctor

Sources of Strength and Wisdom

Edited by
Edvin Schei, Iona Heath,
Peter Dorward, and Caroline Engen

CRC Press
Taylor & Francis Group
Boca Raton London New York

CRC Press is an imprint of the
Taylor & Francis Group, an **informa** business

Designed cover image: View from Roshven, Western Scotland. Photograph by E. Schei.

First edition published 2026
by CRC Press
2385 NW Executive Center Drive, Suite 320, Boca Raton, FL 33431

and by CRC Press
4 Park Square, Milton Park, Abingdon, Oxon, OX14 4RN

CRC Press is an imprint of Taylor & Francis Group, LLC

ISBN: 978-1-032-97334-0 (hbk)
ISBN: 978-1-032-97333-3 (pbk)
ISBN: 978-1-003-59329-4 (ebk)

DOI: 10.1201/9781003593294

Typeset in Bembo
by Apex CoVantage, LLC

The Open Access version of this book was supported by the Norwegian Directorate for Higher Education and Skills, and by University of Bergen.

Contents

Foreword

Arthur W. Frank

These remarkably candid, forthcoming chapters show doctors struggling with one of the first lessons I learned as a professional medicine watcher. Being a physician is not a way to live a normal human life. Doctors see more of life, but their work carries the risk of making them less human.

My first research placement when I started doctoral study in 1970 was to observe in the emergency department of Yale-New Haven Hospital. I remember leaving the hospital very late at night. As I walked past the admissions desk, a man was telling the clerk that he'd been shot. I looked down at his pants and saw what I took to be blood. I thought to myself, if he'd come in several hours earlier, I'd have been interested in following his case. Then I walked out. Even now I think about what just eight hours had turned me into: how I could walk past a human drama as if blood stains were coffee he'd spilled on himself. And I hadn't even been *practising* medicine, only watching, though that too takes practice.

I have watched medicine as an ethnographer with academic stakes in the game, as a patient whose stakes were personal, all too briefly as a visiting clinician on a hospital family-therapy team, occasionally as a bioethicist, and in all these roles, as a writer asking myself the question this book addresses: What is a "good doctor"?

That question elicits a complementary one, which would call for another book: What is a good patient? I am convinced these questions each require the other, because just as a good doctor enables their patient to be a best version of themselves in conditions that risk bringing out the worst, a good patient enables their doctor to be good. The good doctor and the good patient are another chicken-and-egg relationship: Neither comes first, and each creates the possibility of the other. Yet their intimate mutuality is often neglected; each feels apart from the other, disconnected.

When I think about the good doctor, most of the scenes that I flash back to involve being the patient myself. Those scenes have common characteristics. The first is that it isn't what the doctor said—often the words themselves would, in a different context, be flat and even cliché. What made the words matter was the timing of when they were said and an indescribable quality of how they were said. While part of my mind was telling me this was probably a line the doctor used repeatedly, I experienced this person talking to me in the unique here and now of that moment. Actors talk about being able to "sell" a line, which is an awful metaphor but it gets at what I'm trying to describe. How to sell a line? By letting it speak itself as an un-self-conscious expression of who you are; in other words, by meaning it.

Institutional medical practice often distracts physicians from such un-self-conscious, I/thou ways of relating to patients. The phrase "standard of care" has always struck me as badly worded: If actions are based on a *standard*, then they don't fit my understanding of *care*. Care is non-standard specificity of attention to this unique person. A standard of care categorizes the patient and treats them as an instance of that category. Any relationship between persons is subordinated to the standard. Care as I mean it might offer the same treatment, but the good doctor knows how to make it an *offering* to a patient who, in receiving it, feels recognized as distinctive.

Picking up on what makes any individual distinctive isn't usually that hard, although the institutional conditions in which physicians often encounter their patients—stripped of their own clothes and possessions, their lives reduced to what's on a screen—makes being a good doctor more difficult. These days, more of the doctors who diagnose and prescribe for me remain anonymous, unseen in person. For them I exist only on their computer screens, and they exist for me in what tests and medications they order. They help me in ways I appreciate, but I can't call them good doctors. I'm not sure what to call them.

How much about the patient's non-medical life does the good doctor need to know? I've written about and taught what is called *narrative medicine*. Yet I realize that in my experiences as a patient, my good doctors often didn't know much about me. What counted was how they somehow expressed a recognition that there was much more about me, and they might potentially be interested but we had other business at hand, pressing concerns. The narrative felt recognized and so could be left unsaid.

The unsaid is another potential book topic. The good doctor is able to give patients a vocabulary that they need to become able to talk about their illnesses. But the good doctor does not impose a narrative on their patients' experiences. Imposing a narrative includes marking a beginning, defining what counts in the actions that follow from that beginning, and specifying a preferred ending. People need narratives to give their lives a sense of order, and most people don't know how to talk about themselves in the strange new world of being an ill body in a medical setting. Narrative guidance is needed. Guiding without imposing requires tact, a word that should be used more often in medicine: Is doing such-and-such *tactful*?

The good doctors in my life had a way of bringing me out of my not usefully emotional fantasies of what illness was doing to my life, so that I could focus on what could be done about illness. Maybe that's part of William Osler's famous call for equanimity in medical practice. It's a fine balance, how the doctor projects recognizing what's at stake for the patient and projects having their own stake in that patient's life but also comes across as watching from somewhere slightly outside. At best that stance allows the patient to find their own space outside the obsessive preoccupation that illness can become. Phrases attempting to describe this balance end up with oxymorons like detached concern. I wonder whether phrases describing good doctoring need to be oxymoronic or else they are not true. The best writing in these chapters, at least for me, evokes the doctor's ambivalence about whether they've got the engagement/detachment balance right within their practice.

Practice is a word we might do well to get back to using more. Physicians used to join or open a practice; now they get jobs. Practising involves learning, always wanting to learn more. One aspect of learning is the specifically medical stuff of diagnosis and treatment, but that does not set the good doctor apart. The aspect of greater concern in this book—what I think the *art* of medicine involves and what patients sincerely thank their doctors for—is wanting to learn how this patient whose face I see feels about their life, including but not limited to how their symptoms and prognosis affect that life. If the doctor is genuinely curious, then we patients feel treated as fellow human persons who matter to each other. That curiosity can take the form of only one question in any visit; less can actually be more.

What, then, do I most need in order to be a good patient who enables my doctor to be good? Can my doctor help me to articulate and thus confront my fears, because they are confident they can open themselves to fear without being sucked into it? Can my doctor realize how much else besides illness matters to me in my life and accept that our priorities won't always match, because a good doctor has always accepted being only one of the characters on the stage of my life? Can my doctor model in their responsiveness to me the contradiction that the world does care about me—that I truly matter—but the world also has to move on and I should take comfort in knowing it will move on?

As I get older and accumulate doctors at an increasing rate, the question I ask myself about each new doctor is this: Can they be the one whom I want to someday tell me, with nuanced certainty, that this is how I am going to die? The good doctor will be able to give me that message so that I can receive it as a gift. They will balance sadness with reality and thus enable me to remain, even then, curious about my life in all its aspects and narrator of the story of this life. Can this doctor accept my reciprocal gift of enabling them to vicariously encounter their own mortality and thus become less alone, less afraid?

Arthur W. Frank is a Professor Emeritus at the University of Calgary, Canada. His best-known books are *At the Will of the Body*, a memoir of his own critical illnesses, and *The Wounded Storyteller*, a study of how people narrate illness experience and the force of witness. He is a Fellow of the Royal Society of Canada and winner of the 2016 Lifetime Achievement Award from the Canadian Bioethics Society. He can be reached at arthurwfrank@gmail.com and https://arthurwfrank.wordpress.com.

Preface

What Kind of Book Is This? Words of Welcome from the Editors

The authors of this book are all doctors. Cumulatively, we have a great deal of clinical experience. We come from Norway, the United Kingdom, Canada, the Netherlands, and the United States. Some of us are older; some are well-known academics. Others are young, in their first years as doctors: clinicians, researchers, and educators.

We love and esteem our profession, but we are worried.

Medicine seeks to serve and protect the highest values in life. It strives to engage with suffering and mitigate it. We believe that there can be no more noble a task than that.

But we doctors don't always recognize this suffering when we meet it. Sometimes we lack the skill or time or motivation to engage with it when it is presented to us. We scarcely even see it in ourselves. Without that seeing, that recognition, and that knowledge, those vastly effective tools we doctors wield will have no grip.

In this book, we offer ways of being that we believe can help us: learners, educators, clinicians, and patients. We don't naïvely suggest that we can "solve" things: those complex, systemic challenges with roots far beyond medicine itself—but we want to show that there are many diverse and under-explored ways of responding to the hard realities of modern health care. There are sources of strength and wisdom out there. We need to seek them out. We need them all.

Relationship skills and creative collaboration are essential in healing, education, and care but are often neglected in medical education. Some chapters in the book depict or allude to events that took place in two 4-day symposia, one in Rosendal in Norway in 2022, the other in Roshven in Scotland in 2023. Both meetings were dedicated to exploring whether there is such a thing as "The Right Stuff of Medicine" and, if so, what that thing might be.

All authors participated in at least one of the symposia and decided together to create a book based on those experiences. The seminars offered a frame in which we chose to challenge ourselves to step outside conventional "medical knowledge" and deepen our understanding of what people need in sickness and suffering by using our own experiences of vulnerability, our own sources of strength and wisdom. Two of the chapters offer detailed accounts of those events, attempting to write not only the *what* but also possible *hows* of a medical philosophy aiming for change.

Unlike many academic books, this one is a mix of literary genres—dialogues, personal narratives, philosophical arguments, academic prose, clinical vignettes, poetic imagery. This is deliberate. We think that the ability to perceive human problems and plan wise action is hampered when scientific language becomes so dominant that it overshadows other ways of understanding. Medicine needs emotional, narrative, and aesthetic approaches to knowledge and compassion.

If you read the chapters of this anthology in sequential order (or even if you choose your own order), you may have a surprising experience. Bon voyage!

The Editors
Edvin Schei
Iona Heath
Peter Dorward
Caroline Engen

Editors

Edvin Schei

Professor, Section for General Practice, Department of Global Public Health and Primary Care, University of Bergen, Norway

I was, long ago, a critical medical student who hoped in vain that medicine would teach me about people and make me wiser. Slowly, learning from my patients, I found my way as a family doctor, a teacher of medical students, a researcher in medical education, and an advocate of human connection in medicine. I have been a visiting scholar at Boston University, McGill University in Montreal, and Maastricht University. I have learned that medicine, and patients, profit from philosophy, friendliness, humour, and honesty.

Iona Heath

Retired General Practitioner and Past President of the Royal College of General Practitioners, UK

I worked as a general practitioner in a deprived inner-city area of London for almost 35 years. It was an amazing place to work, and I learnt almost everything I know from the courage and endurance of my patients and from colleagues from across the world but perhaps especially from Scandinavia. I discovered that the work of general practice has such an astonishing breadth that reading almost any book, fiction or non-fiction, has something to teach us about the human condition that is relevant to our work. Reading taught me to write, and writing has helped me to think.

Peter Dorward

General Practitioner, NHS Education for Scotland, UK

I am a family physician and medical teacher based in Edinburgh, Scotland. I have a long interest in the intersections of medicine, philosophy, and literature and talk and write extensively on this subject. I am the author of *The Human Kind, A Doctor's Stories from the Heart of Medicine* (Bloomsbury, 2018).

Caroline Engen

Neuro-SysMed, Haukeland University Hospital, Bergen; Centre for the Study of the Sciences and the Humanities, University of Bergen; and Division of Psychiatry, Haukeland University Hospital, Bergen, Norway

I trained as a cancer researcher before turning to psychiatry and a scholarly path in the philosophy of medicine. This path continues to shape both my clinical work and academic inquiry and has taught me to see suffering not only as something to be known and treated but as something that reveals. My work largely focuses on epistemological and ethical dimensions of contemporary medicine.

Contributors

J. Donald Boudreau
Scholar at the Institute of Health Sciences Education, McGill University, Canada
I have been a general practitioner and a lung specialist. I have practised in a high-resource country (Canada) and a low-resource country (Nicaragua), in large cities and rural settings, in non-teaching and teaching hospitals. Having had the privilege to be of service as a physician in these many contexts has been the most meaningful and defining aspect of my life. It has also channelled my research interests. My scholarly contributions to the profession have focused on the personhood—or the "being"—of learners and physicians.

Knut Eirik Eliassen
Associate Professor, Section for General Practice, Department of Global Public Health and Primary Care, University of Bergen, Norway
I am a general practitioner by profession and by heart. After 20 years of clinical work, I am now foremost an educator focusing on medical education and research as well as clinical family practice, medical uncertainty, and decision making. I am invested in faculty development, not least in increasing supervisor competency among the clinical supervisors at the GP offices.

Ronald M. Epstein
Professor of Family Medicine, Oncology and Medicine, American Cancer Society Clinical Research Professor; and Co-director, Research Division, Departments of Family Medicine and Medicine, and Wilmot Cancer Center, University of Rochester Medical Center, Rochester, New York
I am a family physician, palliative care physician, researcher, teacher, mentor, and writer and have devoted my professional life to defining the qualities of mindful practitioners, improving communication in clinical settings, and promoting health professionals' self-awareness and flourishing.

Lara Kesseler

GP Trainee, NHS Education for Scotland, UK

I was at the time of writing a trainee general practitioner (family doctor). Since then, I have completed training and have been taking the first steps as a GP but also taken time to travel, to explore the world outside of medicine, and perhaps to take some of these experiences with me into my future practice.

John Launer

GP Educator and Writer, London; Honorary Lifetime Consultant, Tavistock Clinic London; Visiting Professor, Anglia Ruskin University Faculty of Health Sciences; Honorary Associate Clinical Professor, University College London School of Medicine; Lead Training Programme for Educational Innovation, NHS England (London); and Honorary President, Association of Narrative Practice in Healthcare

My background is as a graduate in English literature, then becoming a doctor, family physician, and family therapist. Since mid-career, I have spent most of my time as a medical educator and writer, promoting the application of narrative ideas and skills to everyday healthcare.

Karl Erik Müller

Registrar in Infectious Diseases, Drammen Hospital, Vestre Viken Hospital Trust; Researcher at Department of Clinical Science, Faculty of Medicine, University of Bergen; and Co-director of Vestre Viken Airway Infections Research Group, Norway

Before entering medical school, I earned a degree in economics. During my medical studies, I discovered two strong passions. The first was for the natural sciences, which led me to conduct research in parasitology and molecular biology, taking me to renowned laboratories in Brazil. The second was rooted in the humanities—I was actively involved in research groups focusing on medical philosophy, medical education, and clinical communication. This dual interest has remained with me throughout my medical journey. As I continue my training to become a specialist in infectious diseases, I remain engaged in research, now with a stronger focus on clinical studies. I'm also dedicated to supporting younger colleagues during their foundation year, guiding reflective group sessions to help them grow professionally and personally.

Margot de Rijke

General Practitioner, Municipality of Rælingen, Norway

I am a junior doctor who has recently established my own practice in family medicine. As a medical student, I became interested in medical teaching and patient communication. As a young doctor, I have become greatly aware of the moral stress we as medical professionals are put under. My road of learning is still long, but I am finding strength and wisdom along the way and am optimistically implementing these in my own practice.

Victoria Schei

Solli District Psychiatric Centre (DPS), Bergen; and Department of Anaesthesia and Intensive Care, Haukeland University Hospital, Bergen, Norway

I graduated from medical school in 2021 and am now specializing in psychiatry. My internship in a medium-sized hospital inspired me to write a piece about the harsh working conditions of junior doctors, which went viral. After a brief period as a general practitioner, I found my place in psychiatry. Here, I learn to become a psychotherapist, under compassionate guidance from specialists, while standing in the front line of acute psychiatry. For me, being a doctor is more than following the algorithms; it requires my whole self.

Eivind Alexander Valestrand

Department of Global Public Health and Primary Care, University of Bergen; and Intern at Akershus University Hospital, Norway

Once, as a child and teenager, I was a patient—dependent on doctors to guide me through life-threatening illness with their knowledge and care.

Then, as a medical student, I had to find a way to use that past to connect with patients, even as it often drew me inward. That was made harder by a medical culture that seemed to overlook the lived experiences of those it served. Now, I am a father of three joyful, energetic kids, deep into medical residency. I'm learning, growing, and dreaming—of a future in medicine shaped by humour, kindness, and meaning.

Lizzie Wastnedge

Clinical Lecturer, Centre for Reproductive Health, University of Edinburgh; and GP Registrar, NHS Education for Scotland, Edinburgh, UK

I am a trainee in general practice and an avid reader and hill runner. I chose a career in general practice because I value the power of stories as both methods of communication and as tools for understanding and transforming. I am currently undertaking a PhD looking at understanding pregnancy planning, where I am exploring epistemology in relation to medical practice and how as a clinician and a researcher I can draw together my biomedical education and my curiosity about people to ultimately evoke change.

1

Beginning

Peter Dorward

> "*Nel mezzo cammin di nostra vita mi ritrovai per una selva oscura.*"
> "In the mid-point of the journey of my life I found myself lost in a dark forest."
>
> **(Dante, *Inferno*)**

Sometimes in medicine, even for someone quite established in their career, even for someone with many years of service, a person can find themselves suddenly lost.

It is as if, momentarily, you have no bearings. No map, no sense of destination, no clear sense of origin. It is as if you have woken suddenly from a deep and dreamless sleep, disorientated. Imagine! Confronted suddenly with your loneliness, a sense perhaps of purposelessness, that nightmarish feeling of having *lost* something. Imagine, a feeling of having been beguiled or deceived, enthralled or even trapped. Imagine, lost, being confronted by the ghost of your younger self, who asks you questions like *How did you end up like that? And why? Why do you keep doing whatever it is you're doing?*

Those kinds of questions you might once have asked of your own parents, if you dared, are now asked of you.

Sometimes we doctors can be afflicted by bad feelings. Sometimes we, whose purpose once seemed so clear and obvious, can find ourselves snared in despair or nihilism.

Yet how much more intense must that feeling be, if it comes, when it comes, for younger people—students, or juniors! And how much more serious!

DOI: 10.1201/9781003593294-1 1

These are my thoughts, anyway, one morning, a couple of years ago, as I startle awake from what seems to have been a dangerously protracted daydream.

Winter of 2022, or thereabouts, south-east Scotland, and I, the doctor, am running late. I'm feeling rather tired, which is dispiriting, because it's still only half nine in the morning and there's a long day ahead. And I'm prone to losing valuable minutes of my day in existential introspection—a habit which is getting somewhat out of control, and frankly a bit of a downer with my colleagues. There have been murmurings. I sense them. So:

I have a child outside, a patient with her parents, waiting to be seen. I need to get a move on.

I'm only five minutes late. I think that that is well within the range of what is acceptable. In fact, I can probably fit in the re-authorization of 12 routine prescriptions before turning my attention to this child, whom I don't believe to be significantly unwell—I'd still only be ten or so minutes late, and that great untouched list of minor administrative tasks daunts me so, grinds me down, always, still.

So maybe I can file some more letters, some more test results.

To be more accurate, I only b*elieve* that this child, waiting outside, is unlikely to be ill—in truth you never *actually* know for sure. You can never quite relax. It's easy to be wrong. Every day in life you take these tiny gambles.

I remember a child whom I saw, about 45,000 patients or so before this, a toddler, presenting just like this, just as innocuously, her mother seeming quite unconcerned over the phone—who turned out to be *very* ill. I was a young GP then. I remember the livid pallor of the child's skin, the bruises, the dummy she didn't have the energy to suck on, the trail of dribble on her cheek, the sunken half-closed eyes, the look on the child's mother's face, when she saw the look on *my* face.

That was a long time ago. It's the first time I've thought of that child in a long time. That child survived, but only just. The trace of her memory survives, engraved in me.

But *this* child, today's child, is five years old, and nothing in the story, when I spoke to them 20 minutes ago, had worried me.

Yet I still said, *"Yes! Fine! Come straight up, I've got time,"* knowing that, in truth, I have little time.

You see, I can remember what it is to be the parent of a five year old whom you believe *might* be unwell. How that worry corrodes. So, really, it is for the child's parents that I have agreed urgently to have them bring this child up. It is the child's *parents* who are really, in this case, my patient.

Or possibly it is the memory of my own younger self that drives me: the father, 25 years ago, who would have been so grateful to a doctor, who was prepared to drop everything to attend to *my worry*. Maybe I just want to be *that* doctor. Perhaps that is what is really motivating me—the appeal of acting like a good human being. I do still remember that doctor. We called her out one night, young, worried parents, in the middle of the night, on account of some trivia. How gracious she was, though tired.

But now I'm seven and a half minutes late. And I need to stop losing myself down memory holes.

I stand, abruptly. I leave my room to collect my patient. Opposite the door to my office is a mirror. I catch a glimpse of myself in that mirror as I leave.

This blurred reflected self I catch—his tired, rushed look.

"Lilly!"

I call Lilly through. Five years old, a princess in pink, a unicorn clutched in her right hand, a smile on her face, her slightly flushed face.

Lilly leaps to her feet. She responds well to the smile of welcome that I wear. A habit—a good one—cultivated over many years. I wave to the child, who half-waves back, and her mother says, "say hello to the doctor, Lilly!" and Lilly says "hello!"

And I think, Ach, Lilly's going to be just fine.

★   ★   ★

Last night I met a stranger. Two strangers, both doctors. One Norwegian, one Canadian. A Zoom call.

The Canadian had read something I had written a couple of years previously and liked it. A friend of a friend of a friend—a chain of people whom I respected—had handed my text between them, and now this person wanted, out of the blue, to speak with me. I am flattered by this attention.

I don't at this point know what it is that these two want from me. They sent me an email—then another. The first went to "junk." Something about "values." The "core values of medicine." What that might mean.

Sometimes, I have learned, stumbling along as you do in the forest of your life, picking out those half-marked traces that mark your way, you meet people, if you're lucky, who might suggest better, clearer routes. The suggestions these rare, good folk make are often rather subtle. Understated. It matters to notice them.

So, two men on a Zoom. My age, more or less. Perhaps a little older. One nods to the other. *Begin*.

"There is a lot of suffering in the world." Begins the Norwegian. *Edvin*, is his name. "And a lot of alienation. In us. The doctors whose job it is to recognize and mitigate it."

He seems at first rather solemn, Edvin, but the light is bad, and so is the sound. Appearances can deceive, especially over Zoom.

"There is a persistent sense of dislocation. Between our calling, our purpose—and our actions. It's as if we have cultivated this inability to behave in the world in accordance with our values. Our best values."

The Canadian, Tom, nods, grunts, as doctors do.

"And we, healers, risk becoming unable to respond to the call of suffering. Unable to hear its voice, or understand the language that it speaks in. The contrast between the ostensible nobility of our calling and the reality of our day to day practice has become *very* great."

Do I warm to any of this? Is the world not full enough already of powerful people setting the rest to right? This all seems a bit . . . grandiose. *"The voice of suffering. The nobility of our calling."* I don't know, frankly.

But then, the work of any of us might seem grandiose if so described. From the nursing auxiliary with a dampened cloth who brings some final dignity to the recently dead before the dead one's relative comes to say goodbye, to the surgeon who breathes a momentary prayer, humble, before he makes his cut—there *is* such grandeur in our work; it's everywhere, if we care to see it.

And I, I silently concede, often find it hard to behave in the world according to good values. To *any* values. You see, often I'm too tired, stressed, and distracted. And uncertain, truth be told, what these *core values* might even be. And where they come from.

Tom picks it up.

"We're bringing a group of doctors together to explore this theme. Call it, for now, 'The Right Stuff of Medicine.' We wondered whether you might be interested in joining us? Would this be your kind of thing?"

★ ★ ★

This *is* my kind of thing.

The practice of medicine, I believe, is laced with unexamined philosophical questions and assumptions. By and large, we doctors are untrained and unused to thinking about them. If we can't see them, these questions, for what they are—if we are blind to them—then we are fundamentally lost. Lost in a dark forest.

These questions might include:

- *What is the nature of suffering?*
- *With what language does it speak?*
- *Does medicine understand this language of suffering?*
- *Can technological medicine, by its nature, respond to the needs of the suffering person? And if not, why not?*
- *And if it can't, how could it?*
- *And if it doesn't, or can't, what effect does that have on doctors and their patients?*
- *And if we were to take these kinds of questions seriously, what would that mean for us, our practice, our training, our way of being?*

All of which Edvin seems to be concerned with. And as he talks, I'm thinking I've been worrying about this kind of stuff my whole life—but lacked the proper tools to think about it.

And I'm thinking again about this feeling, this sense that has been growing in me lately, but has always been there, of being lost.

"The idea is this: We meet together. Fourteen of us, more or less. A diverse group of doctors, for a few days, to consider these questions and ways to respond as clinicians, as educators, as leaders, as individuals. What are the core values of our craft? What are the major threats to these values? What tools may be required to meet these threats, and survive, and thrive? Place matters. It needs to be somewhere far away from home or work, somewhere beautiful. We have some ideas.

"The meeting will involve the sharing of stories and experience, workshops, talks, presentations, walking, swimming, humour, music, the sharing of art or literature, the preparation of food and the sharing of it. We will consider whether we might participate in future such groups, and if so, how? All the processes and materials are generated by the group."

A pause.

"And we may want to see whether a book emerges from these meetings."

This, then, is that book:

1   **Beginning**

A doctor, lost somewhere in the middle of his life, receives a call from a stranger. An invitation to join a weeklong medical seminar, spring time, in Norway. Difficult questions are to be explored concerning the nature of medicine, the nature of suffering, and the kind of knowledge we may need to understand these things. What they will come to call "The Right Stuff of Medicine." They will range freely, over difficult terrain, sometimes coming too close to the edge, sometimes almost falling off. There will be difficulties, disagreement, conflict perhaps—but at least it's springtime, at least the birds will sing.

2   **I'm Dreading This**

Do *you* still remember it? Your first day on shift?

In this, a new doctor experiences her first, traumatic day at work. Nothing in her training has quite prepared her for this dreadful paradox: that you can be a person who is kind, skilled, and compassionate—a humane moral agent—or you can know your stuff, do the job, and get through the shift. It seems hard to be both, and impossible if you're on your own. There will be blood.

3   **Framing the Problem: Suffering and Knowing in the World of Things**

Two clinicians explore the same problem from different perspectives—one from the tradition of critical philosophy, the other from a general practitioner's clinic.

The problem is this: that suffering is subjective, personal, and unique. Medicine is technical, scientific, and objective—it makes *things* out of people—it has to. Subjective suffering and objective medicine don't share a natural language. They conflict. This can lead to confusion and more suffering. It might also generate new ways forward, new ways of knowing.

4   **When Death Comes to Work**

A young doctor's identity is shaken to its core by the unexpected visitation of death.

It affects us; it affects us over and over again. Perhaps it shouldn't, but it does, always.

5   **Medicine: We Make It; It Makes Us**

What then *is* our identity? We contain multitudes. This chapter explores how doctors are formed. How medical identity, in turn, affects those forces that make us what we are.

6   **Levels of Experience**

We *all* suffer, even doctors. Especially tired ones; sad ones; young, frightened ones; or old, complacent ones. In this, two clinicians, one new and younger, one older and more experienced, write about patient suffering, doctor suffering, how these forms of suffering interact, and how they determine outcomes.

7   **Steps toward Deep Listening**

It's harder to treat a person as a thing if you have first known them as a person. In this, an older doctor finds that the capacity to *listen* is more than a skill, but an attribute, deeply moral in its nature, that must be learned, treasured, and maintained. Without it, we cannot bridge that hazardous gap between people and things.

8   **Your Everyday—My Once in a Lifetime**

Here, a doctor experiences the consequences of this firsthand. What it's like to be on the receiving end of the casual harms of medicine.

9 Dialogue and Healing

In this, the deeper *how* of listening is discussed. What you might hear, what you might learn, what you might do with the stories that might emerge. The transforming skills of narrativity in medicine are explored, and through them we glimpse new ways forward.

10 Attending to the Unsaid: On Knowing, Care, and Voice

What we know, what we think we know, what we know we *need* to know—it is all already mapped out. How do we progress when we have reached the limit of the territory of words?

In this, an eruption of uncertainty. Joy, chaos, frivolity, song, and Nepalese gongs.

We healers have our souls too, unknowable, beyond words. How do we nurture them? How do we keep ourselves going, to carry on with this, our burden, our carrying?

11 I'll Take It with Me When I Go

A simple, powerful, worked example of the above . . . Try it out.

12 Alienation, Resonance, and the Formation of Physicians

- Who am I now, if I'm not to be that hero, who cured you when you were sick?
- What am I, if my touch no longer heals?
- What have I, if I have lost the gift of kindness?
- Who will hear me if I've forgotten how to listen?
- Medicine is beset now with despair, grief, loss of meaning, anger, bitterness, disconnection, burnout.
- What have we become?
- And what *could* we be?

13 Second Thoughts—Reflections on Early Medical Career Experiences

The long, slow journey towards mastery.

A little pushback here—this, doctoring, was always going to be hard. A bit of a slog at times. It needs to be. It needs to hurt a little. It's worth it.

14 Wisdom in Medical Practice

Phronesis, or practical wisdom. In this, a physician considers—so, *given all of this, what does it take in this age to be wise?*

I'm Dreading This

Victoria Schei

"I'm dreading this." An unwelcome thought, coming, for the first time, unbidden, wholly unexpected.

It's mid-afternoon, and I am headed to the medium-size hospital where I've got a job as an intern. The job application process was long, competitive, and arduous. Thirteen places, 657 applicants. *I am lucky*, I tell myself, ignoring the slight anxiety that is making me walk faster than usual.

As I am approaching the gloomy grey concrete building, I guess I am as ready as I ever could be, my bag prepped with a stethoscope, a pen, a name tag, and meticulously selected food and snacks to get me through the 18 hours on call.

Just yesterday, I was on a tour of this emergency room. My "orientation visit." Irony. It feels like years ago. We were 13 interns. My new colleagues were mostly young women like me. The five guys seemed to have already formed a bond, giving high fives and, from the looks of it, making plans during orientation week.

From what I've been told by the previous interns, the emergency room will be my second home. The tour was given by the head nurse of the department, a polished woman in her mid–40s, dressed in a skirt suit and stiletto heels.

Only minutes into the tour, a guy with a black Nike cap pretended to press the code button with an exaggerated hand gesture, looking over at his new best friends who were laughing and trying to hide it. Mrs Stiletto Heel shot him a stern look.

DOI: 10.1201/9781003593294-2

"You push that button, and the cardiac team will all leave their patients and come running. This is the real world, and you will look very stupid in it." I felt a glow of pleasure that I am not proud of.

She introduced us to a dozen on-call nurses dressed in scrubs in their break room, eating and chatting and laughing. Some were smiling at us; the older, more tired ones, more critically—sizing us up.

Our group of interns followed Mrs Stiletto Heel through the newly refurbished corridors of the emergency room that contrasted with the dilapidated exterior of the building. We were beeped through modern doors and peeked into similar-looking rooms—the biolab, the storage room, the linen room. They would soon become familiar.

I passed the nurses' break room after the tour was over and heard them laughing.

"Yeah well—they get younger each year." Sigh. "Like lambs to the bloody slaughter." More laughter. I met the gaze of Mrs Stiletto Heel, who saw me overhearing. I left quickly.

★   ★   ★

The sun is shining through the windows of the hospital hall which I am rapidly traversing on my way to the dressing rooms. I hear my stomach making whale-like sounds—not sure whether it's something I ate or nerves—but I need to find a toilet.

After changing into scrubs, I look at myself in the mirror. *I have studied for so many years. I'm ready, I can do this.*

On my way from the dressing rooms to the emergency room, I think about the dinner I had with my friend, Maria, and her grandmother yesterday. Maria comes from this town; we used to sing in the same student choir. She is one of the few people I know here.

Her grandmother showed great interest yesterday when I answered her polite question about my occupation and said I was a doctor. The old woman approached me and showed me her right knee, covered in grey tights. "Doesn't it look swollen to you? Here, feel it," she said, leading my hand to her knee. I felt obliged to squeeze it lightly. The knee did not look or feel swollen. "It has been so painful for so long," she said with a worried tone.

"Oh, that must be bothersome. Did anything happen?" I asked out of duty.

"No, but it *has* to be something. What if I'm walking around with a fracture or an excruciate ligament? My friend had one of those!"

She went on to tell me about a rude intern she had met yesterday because her general practitioner was on sick leave.

"That young thing looked like she had barely finished high school. When I asked to get referred to an MRI, she said no, and that I had to try physical therapy! Can you believe how rude she was? Who is *she* to decide?"

I did not have the energy to enter the discussion. I nodded, even though it sounded like the intern had given decent advice.

"I'm sorry, I know you are an intern, but I just find it hard to trust you young doctors," the grandmother said. "I want an experienced doctor, preferably a man. Tell me, why *do* they put the new ones in the emergency room? I have never understood that system."

I find myself envying Maria, who works in marketing, has an office job with a good salary, and is not responsible for sorting out old ladies' bodily complaints, or for knowing what to do in life-or-death situations. *I will be, in about two minutes.* The anxiety hits me. *But I do have someone to call, so it will be fine. Right?*

★ ★ ★

The doors to the emergency room swing open as I beep my card. The contrast from the quiet hall outside to the busy waiting room is striking. It is filled with people of all ages—an old woman on crutches, a mother holding a crying baby, a five year old impatiently running around, a pale man in his 20s puking into a bag. Beeping sounds from different directions cut the air, and a digital display shows a blinking "room 5" in red letters. People dressed in green and white scrubs rush past me holding papers and talking on phones.

I find my way to the doctors' on-call room. Around eight white coats are sitting at their computers writing intensely. It seems like no one is noticing me, except Nike cap guy from yesterday, who is looking quite different—untidy, pale, and haggard.

"There you are," he says. "I'm Eric. Victoria, right?"

He hands me the phone and the pager quicker than I am prepared for.

"It's been . . . *so* busy today. The phone never stopped ringing. There are eight patients waiting, I just haven't had the time to get through them all." His eyes are red. *Is his lower lip slightly twitching?*

"And there are more coming in," he says, pointing to the screen.

He is referring to a long list of patients who are on their way to the hospital. I see names in green, yellow, and red, indicating the severity of their condition.

"Oh, and there are three patients on the fifth floor that you need to check on. Apparently, an old woman with lung cancer has a dropping blood pressure. One of them needs to have an arterial blood gas."

"Aha," I say slowly, as I try to take it all in.

Nike cap logs off the computer and gives me a look as if he feels sorry for me. "Well, good luck! Hope it calms down," he says, picks up his backpack, and leaves.

All of these patients, waiting just for me. Okay, I can do this. Just be focused and structured, one thing at a time.

The eight patients waiting are marked with different symptoms on my screen—"acute abdominal pain," "rectal bleed," "back fracture and possible COVID," "femoral neck fracture," "dislocated shoulder," and so on. Their waiting time is counting upwards—7 hours, 46 minutes and 32, 33, 34 seconds, it says below the name of a 76-year-old man with a back fracture. He has a foreign name, I notice.

A nurse enters the room and starts talking, snapping me out of my train of thought.

"Who is responsible for the man in room 7? He has been waiting for almost eight hours to see a doctor, and he is in a lot of pain," she says with a sharp tone, looking around. No one responds.

"I am," I say, clearing my throat. "I just started my shift, but I will look into it and see him as soon as possible. Let me just get an overview."

"Are you one of the new interns? You need to see him straight away," she shoots quickly. I nod submissively.

"Two minutes, I promise."

I quickly browse his referral and note some key points: "Fell on the ice this morning"—"fever and coughing"—"needs an Iranian translator." Vitals are fine. Has only received paracetamol and ibuprofen through the day.

I get up and head into the hallway, looking for room 7, trying to ignore all the other tasks that are making it hard to focus. He is isolated because of the suspected COVID infection. I put on the yellow suit as I learned in the mandatory e-course yesterday, finishing with a tight mask and visor to protect my face from any virus.

I enter the room, introduce myself with my name and title—already my visor is steaming up . . .

"برای من یک دکتر مناسب بیاور" the patient says, with some anger.

I had forgotten. About the translator. He is sweating, and from his expression he is in pain.

His son answers for him. "Can you give him something? Maybe morphine?" His expression is desperate.

"Yes, I will give him something, let me just examine him," I say firmly.

The mask drills into my cheeks as I try to get a history. The man has no chance of understanding and is, from the looks of it, just getting angrier.

Taking an arterial blood gas—a procedure I have only practised during training—turns out to be hopeless through gloves and with the patient's sudden movements. I try twice, then give up, and let the eager male nurse who has been standing in the background give it a go. As the blood enters the syringe and he succeeds, he gives me a triumphant look.

Questions about painkillers interrupt me while I try to examine the patient, coming from both the son and the nurse. I realise I have to do something. I hear myself saying to the nurse to administer 2.5 mg of morphine IV and to have metoclopramide ready in case of nausea.

As I take off my clammy yellow protection gear afterwards, I feel unsure about the decision of giving him morphine. This did not feel like the consultations I practised in medical school.

I return to the work room. On the computer next to me, a male doctor is typing intently, taking breaks only to dive into the pages of a thick book and take sips of a Diet Coke. I'm guessing he is a resident. He must be about five years older than me. I want to get some reassurance, but at the same time I don't want to interrupt him. *Well, he looks kind, so I'll take the chance.*

"Hey," I start, hesitantly.

He keeps typing for a few seconds, then looks at me. I can tell he is bothered.

"You seem busy, but it's my first shift. Can I ask you something?"

He must have seen my distress. He sighs, gives me a tired smile.

"First shift—don't envy you. What do you need?"

"You are in medical, right? Have you done surgery?"

"Sure," he says, turning back and typing away.

"I just gave a man with back pain morphine. Is 2.5 mg okay?" I say, hoping he is still listening. He pauses.

"Yes, they usually need that, sometimes more. Just as long as his blood pressure and saturation is okay. You know we have a pain protocol for back pain, right?" Wrong—I've never heard of that.

He shows me a sort of guideline for back pain patients, explaining which tests we have to do and the ladder of pain medication preferred by this hospital. I had not done all the tests, I'd jumped straight to morphine—but hey ho, he was in so much pain.

"Show me his radiology," he says, and I am taken aback that he is actually offering to spend time helping me.

"It's a stress fracture," he says, glancing at the dark x-ray of the patient's spine. "He can be sent home, or to a nursing home just to get pain medication for a few days," he says.

The pager interrupts us. Beep beep beep! I look down. CAR ACCIDENT, it says, my body tenses before I have finished reading the words.

"Car accident," I say to him. He understands my confusion.

"Just go to the trauma room, take notes and an arterial blood gas. That is your task. The specialists do the trauma examination," he reassures me. I do as instructed.

The shift continues in a frenzy. At 8 p.m. I realise that I have not been to the toilet or eaten anything. *There will never be a right time. There is no break here.*

I exit the chaotic emergency room—feeling like I am sneaking out—crossing my fingers that the phone will stay silent for just ten minutes. It does.

Back in the on-call room, a blonde woman in her late 30s enters. She's dressed in green scrubs, a paper cap on her head. Red marks around her nose from a face mask reveal she came straight from the operating theatre. I suspect she's my resident on call. *Finally. I have so many questions lined up.*

"You are the intern in surgical, right?" she asks me.

"Yes. Could I just—" I pull up my notebook.

"I'm headed home now. Only call me if there is anything important that you can't solve on your own. You know, necrotising fasciitis, open fractures, that sorta thing. All right, have a good one," she says and vanishes out the door.

I work at high speed for the next hours, my neck tense and cheeks red, going from one patient to the next, frequently interrupted by the phone. Most of the consultations involve containing the frustration of patients or relatives about the time they have waited. I excuse myself again and again, smiling politely while suppressing feelings of bitterness.

In the mini-breaks walking between rooms, I try to build myself up. *I am giving this everything I have. I am working as hard as I can. I cannot do more.*

At four o'clock in the night, I find time to sit down and heat my porridge in the empty break room. The microwave sound is calming. I take a deep breath and let myself sink into the sofa.

Next on my list is a patient in the general surgical department who needs to have his notes done. For him to be officially admitted here, for the paperwork and the reimbursements, it is required that he be examined by a doctor, even though he was transferred directly from another hospital. This formalistic detail is jarring; I am tired.

He's in his mid–40s, but sleeping like a child. I shake him. He looks so tired, and so pissed off. But then again, so am I. I explain the circumstances and bring him to a separate examination room, and in an uninspired way I go through the required list of questions that I have already asked so many patients this night.

"Allergies?"

"No."

"How have your stools been lately? Any blood?"

"No. Can I go to sleep now?"

"Yes soon, I just need to finish this, it's standard procedure. I am sorry you had to wait so long, it was quite busy tonight."

"I can see that. Apparently, I have not been prioritised. Can you explain why you've put me in the corridor?" he says, his eyebrows raised.

"Oh, I didn't have anything to do with that. The hospital is full, the nurses have to put the patients where there is space left. That's just the way it is."

He stands up, and I notice how tall he is.

"Well, please see to it that I get my own room and that I am moved immediately."

Clenching his jaw, he leans forward and takes a step towards me.

"I understand sir, but I am a doctor, so my job is to ensure your medical needs, not to assign rooms. Like I said, I don't have anything to do with the practicalities."

"Do you know who I am?" he says, louder, clenching his fists. "I run an oil rig in Latin America. I have never been put in the hallway of any hospital, and I refuse to accept this treatment. I thought we had a good welfare system in this country, and this is what I get? A girl who doesn't know anything about me, asks all the same questions that I have answered a million times, and who sees me in the middle of the night—and on top of that, a corridor bed?" He stares at my name badge and nods.

Is this for real? Are you going to make this first shift even worse than it already was, you spoiled brat? I am so tired, at least you get to sleep. Please don't sue me. Or hit me.

He steps back, looking a little ashamed.

"Eh, never mind. Just do what you have to do and let me go back to sleep," he says in a milder tone.

"We have finished, so I'll leave you to it. I have other patients waiting. Good night," I say and turn around. Writing up his notes, I make sure to describe his statements in detail.

Next, I receive a call from the orthopaedic department. "We have a young terminal cancer patient with a saturation of 70%. Can you come see him? He has trouble breathing. His sister is here, and she is quite demanding," the nurse says.

In the dark orthopaedic department, lit only by the green exit signs, I hear snoring from several rooms and faint singing from the end of the hall. I locate the on-call room, and the nurse who looks like she expects me.

"He is 22 years old and has an osteosarcoma with metastases to the lungs. He has been worsening during the last couple of days. He is terminal," she says. I appreciate not having to ask for context. *She is a good nurse.*

"Okay. And the sister?" I ask.

"She demands an x-ray of the chest. She's quite upset, understandably."

I quickly scroll through the last notes about the patient. *Stopped all treatment, only palliative medication*, it reads. Written yesterday by a specialist.

The young man's room is filled with a spicy and sweet smell—cinnamon, maybe? It reminds me of backpacking in India when I was a student. The floor is covered in thick blankets. Bending down is a young woman I'm assuming is his sister, muttering prayers. Three middle-aged people are sitting in chairs by the bed. A beautiful woman in her mid-40s I'm assuming is his mother is crying silently in a chair by the window. She seems resigned.

The patient is sitting on his bed, leaning forward. His skin is moist and jaundiced, his eyes half open looking into the back of his skull, only the whites of the eyes showing. His breath is rapid and superficial. With every intake of air, a faint rasping sound escapes, as though the airways are partly obstructed. The scene is making me nauseous.

"Are you the doctor?" His sister jumps up and approaches me.

"He can't breathe, you need to do something!" Her voice is high-pitched and strained; she's holding her hands up as though she is begging me.

I meet her gaze, nod respectfully, and introduce myself as calmly as I can.

I talk to the patient. No reaction. I touch his shoulder, but it is as though he cannot hear me, using the last of his strength to try to breathe.

I have not seen many dying patients, but I have no doubt that this 26 year old is one.

From the corner of my eye, I see the green numbers on the screen showing that his oxygen levels are sinking.

"Saturation is 67%," the nurse says.

"He needs to get an x-ray of the lungs! His lungs are filled with water, you can't just let him . . . drown," his sister says, and starts sobbing.

I feel trapped, but cannot escape.

In despair, I take out my stethoscope and lift the young man's moist shirt up. Even though he doesn't seem able to hear me, I explain that I am going to listen to his lungs. *As if that will help.* The wheezing and crackles are so loud and clear through the stethoscope, it's painful to listen to.

He is dying and I cannot fix that. An x-ray will not help.

My face is clearly showing something—the whole of my body too, but I can't, in the moment, know what that is. I'm *feeling* this huge complex of emotion—sadness—real, felt—for the man, and his family. Some fear. An overwhelming need to *help*, to *get this right. Perhaps,* I think, *this is what they meant, at medical school, when they talked—so much!—about "empathy"?*

I leave the room to think. *I clearly have to do something. But I don't know what.*

"Maybe you will feel better if you call your resident," the nurse says. *I needed to hear that.*

I call my resident, hear the ringing tone. *This situation must qualify to call her.* No answer. I try again. The nurse looks worried and checks the number for me. She tries to call her as well—nothing.

"This needs to be reported," she says. "She *should* be available, it's her job."

You always have someone to call, they said. You have a safety net. Well, where is it? Bloody hell, this job.

I decide I have to break the unwritten rules of hospital life and call the kind medical resident—who isn't technically responsible for orthopaedic patients—but who might be the only one who can help me.

The relief when he answers and agrees to come is strong. We see the patient together, and he assures me the right thing is to do nothing. I thank him and he leaves me to tell the family.

Giving a death message on my first night shift. Welcome to doctoring.

"I am sorry, there is nothing we can do. He is dying. He is already on all the medication we can give. An x-ray will only make him suffer more. Your job is to be here and support him."

I leave the room, feeling changed.

★   ★   ★

After a few hours of light sleep from around 6 to 8 a.m., the morning finally comes. I brush my teeth and groggily head to the morning meeting. *My* surgical resident looks rested and content.

"Calm first night shift?" she snaps at me and holds up her phone.

"No calls—never happened before," she says.

"Well *no*, it was *not* calm and I tried to call you several times," I say, noticing that the lack of sleep is making me less inhibited.

"What? Did you use my landline?"

"What home number?"

"Everyone knows, the resident is at home. You should call me at home!" she says, rolling her eyes.

"Well, no one told me that. You could have said so when you left. It was my first shift. I have been really struggling," I say.

"All the other new interns have figured it out," she says, smug.

I swallow my anger and refer the patients of the night. When I arrive at the terminal patient, I say: "I did not manage to reach my superior, so I had to call the medical resident."

"She didn't know about the home number," the resident says, looking around the room for a response. "Well, at least I got a good night's sleep," she says, blinking. The audience laughs. It reminds me of match night at the Union Bar at Uni—all those happy chaps, gathered in a pack, like dogs.

"You interns have got nothing to complain about," one of the eldest growls at me. "In my time, we didn't have anyone to call at all. I was on call for a whole weekend with no breaks and no one to call." He stretches, theatrically, and yawns.

I feel like I have reached my limit. I recognize the unwelcome feeling of tearing up, but manage to hold it in, reminding myself that it is over now. I hand over the phone and pager to the intern who's on call today.

Soon I can sleep.

★   ★   ★

As I leave the meeting room and enter the hallway, I see Mrs Stiletto Heel, headed in my direction. She, seeing my distress, looks away.

After changing out of scrubs, I walk through the reception of the hospital. Coming from the cafeteria is the sister of the cancer patient. I try to meet her eye. She hurries past, ignoring me.

3

Framing the Problem: Suffering and Knowing in the World of Things

Caroline Engen and Peter Dorward

Caroline: This chapter unfolds through two voices. Not in conversation with each other, exactly. Not friends chatting across a kitchen table. Rather, two presences in dialogue with the same space: the clinical space. One speaks from within—immersed in the daily demands, compromises, and intimacies of practice. The other speaks from without—tracing the contours of the clinical field, theorizing, critiquing, resisting.[1] These voices are *versions* of our own, carrying traces of where we come from, but shaped to amplify and refine, to draw out particular ways of seeing—of knowing. Developed, not as direct representations, but as distinct orientations. These voices do not simply describe medicine. They struggle with it. With what it asks. With what it fails to ask. With what it demands of the ones who suffer— and of those who bear witness to that suffering.

At times the voices echo one another; at others, they pull apart, fray, misalign. Like a doctor and a patient both grappling with disease, each with different knowledge, different language, different stakes, these voices move through and in relation to the clinical space without always seeing it the same way. What emerges between them is not agreement or synthesis, but a space of tension—sometimes even estrangement. A third presence. Not a voice, exactly, but

DOI: 10.1201/9781003593294-3

a residue. A silence. Not a void, but something saturated—with discomfort, misrecognition, things not said. The voices grapple with medicine not as a neutral space, but as a site of ethical intensity—where systems intersect with bodies, where expectations collide with uncertainty, and where suffering is rarely just biological. It is relational. Social. The voices grapple with structures that not only hold but constrain—structures that fracture. The absences it creates. The distortions it produces. This third presence does not articulate itself in words, but in the sense of something missed, something lost, something resisted, something suffered.

And it is this very suffering—existential, relational, social—that has the potential to become a site of knowing. Painful, yes. But also generative. Because it marks the limits of what can be said. Because it reveals a cost: what it costs us when voices aren't heard.

This chapter does not aim to reconcile these perspectives. It does not aim to solve or settle. It aims to stay with the fracture, the discomfort, the ambivalence. It holds out the possibility that by attending to the tensions—rather than smoothing them over—we might access a different kind of knowing. A more situated one. A more human one.

So start with Peter, one morning.

Going to work.

On his bike.

Doubt, Ambiguity, and Reflexivity in the Clinical Space

Peter: Mornings now are cold and full of hazards.

Just a month or two ago I was making this trip in shorts and a T-shirt. Like a teenager, leaping on my bike, accelerating mindless with joy over the dry pavements and pot-holed streets of my home town as the world woke up, the air clean, last night's rain making it look like the world had washed its face, bright and fresh for a new day.

Not like that today though. My back wheel skids a little over wet leaves—my heart skitters—there glistens something in the dark that looks like ice on the road. *Slow down,* I think, *slow down.*

This is my time of day.

The air is frozen and wet, damp air clings to my skin, feels like sweat, though I'm not sweating, yet.

I can see my breath hanging in spirals in the thick air, mingling with traffic smoke.

I reflect, smug, at how clean this form of transport makes me feel, how uncomplicated.

I stop at the killer junction—pause, one foot down on the slippery ground, one on the pedal, wait for the traffic to pass—a bin lorry, a bus, an enormous Volvo built like a SWAT team carrier, just taking the children to school.

This is my time of day. This is when I can think. This is the time of day when I can *feel*, most clearly. This is when I am a thinking body, me, threading my way through traffic, my heart in my mouth, stopping at the lights, or jumping them, if it makes me safer.

This is my time of day. This is when I feel most skilful. Out of breath, heart pumping hard now. Powerful, in a way, though powerless too, constantly at risk, constantly negotiating that risk.

Now I am in balance, I think, as I gather speed into the darkness, this long unlit section of cycle path, grimy with mud, rotten leaves, pools of gathered rain water. Why do I go so very fast? Why do I risk this, this all, knowing what I know, about the transience of life?

I arrive a little early at work, at my clinic. Pause a moment, before going in.

I need to take a breath. I need to have a shower. I need to gather myself, prepare myself for what I need to face, this morning, every working morning.

I keep hidden, private in my heart the memory of that simple balance. A body, alive, taking risks with itself, the joy and solace in that.

I enter the clinical space.

My heart always feels a little heavy at this time. Trepidation. I have done this job for many years, yet still I feel this—on a good day a flicker of joy and anticipation, on a bad day, dread.

The clinical space is a contested space. It is full of passion, tears, laughter, conflict, resolution, violence, peace, hate, love.

It embeds within it technology, history, culture, politics, values, philosophy, knowing, and ignorance.

It contains within it all of us: our experience, our complexity.

It is a space where we encounter the edges of our being.

I think sometimes that I understand less of it now than when I started out.

Sometimes I yearn all day for the thrill and simple risk of my short journey home.

But now, right now, my challenge is this. I must navigate the clinical space.

★   ★   ★

Caroline: An urban landscape. A general practitioner riding his bike. Not just an image, but a real glimpse of what late modern medicine is—and what it demands. What plays out in the small risks of the ride plays out again inside the clinic: a navigation not only of patients and symptoms but of the unstable, shifting spaces that late modernity brings into being.[2]

Clinical spaces are neither fixed nor easily defined. They are hazy, shifting, and multifaceted. Rooted in cultural, social, and institutional norms, clinical spaces do not simply express the "medical"; they also reflect broader social dynamics. In late modernity—under conditions of rapid change, individualization, and reflexivity—clinical spaces evolve at a relentless pace. Shaped by large systemic forces, they come to mirror the features of the societies they emerge from: commercialization, bureaucratization, specialization, and an increasing reliance on technology, quantification, and evidence-based approaches.

These evolving spaces continuously reshape the experiences and identities of the individuals who navigate them, while at the same time also being relentlessly re-created by the ideas, ideals, and practices of those very individuals. For both healthcare recipients and providers, then, navigating clinical spaces means not only addressing medical concerns but also negotiating one's place and identity within them. This negotiation unfolds within a wider web of societal expectations, institutional norms, and power structures. Each clinical encounter becomes a reflection of broader social dynamics, a space where expectations, responsibilities, and both legal and moral obligations are continuously renegotiated. Increasingly—just as in late modern societies more broadly— ideals of autonomy, responsibility, and choice are emphasized. These are not incidental, but core features of the ongoing movement toward individualization.

As in broader society, the integration of technoscience into healthcare is marked by a dynamic interplay between emerging risks and reflexive practices. As scientific and technological developments continue to transform healthcare they raise new social, ethical, and political concerns. The impact of disruptive technologies—such as biotechnologies and information systems—extends far beyond medical practice, reshaping understandings of the human and the humane. Individuals, as Ulrich Beck suggests in his theory of reflexive modernity, do not simply adapt to these changing conditions; they engage with them critically. Many recognize that their actions generate not only control and progress but also harm and risk. Across the healthcare system, diverse stakeholders—providers, recipients, policymakers, researchers, and advocacy groups—participate in an ongoing cycle of reflection and adaptation, continuously examining, critiquing, and reshaping institutions and practices in response to evolving norms, risks, and challenges.

Attention to medicine's role in society has intensified—and so has critical scrutiny of its impact. This growing engagement has exposed deep tensions and unresolved conflicts. Modern medicine is often seen as a force for humanization, a source of moral commitment, a project of emancipation. Yet increasingly, it is also viewed as a source of alienation, a form of oppression—even a contributor to the fragmentation of contemporary life. Medicine and its practitioners are no longer seen only as healers or helpers. In some accounts, they appear as dehumanizers, dominators, agents of colonization. This dual image—medicine as both cure and harm—captures not only the complex and often contradictory role medicine plays in late modern society but also the demands placed on those who practice it: moving through change, balancing nature and technology, holding together individuality and connection, opportunity and risk, knowing and not knowing, freedom and responsibility.

It is from within this ambiguity—from the recognition of unintended harms and the reflexivity they demand—that this chapter begins: with a critical reassessment of medicine's foundations, its tensions, and the responsibility and response-ability of those who practice it.

Fragmentation and Organized Irresponsibility

Peter: It can seem that I, the healer, must occupy this ambiguous, at times, irreconcilable role. On the one hand, companion-guide to the suffering other, on the other, a technician.

Given a straight choice, I know which I prefer.

When I was a child—in common with many children—I always ate first the food on my plate that I liked least. Save the best for last! These childhood dispositions run deep.

My first task of the working day, before I let myself do anything that I actually *like*, is to reissue lists of drugs requested by patients. The list is always very long. The task is morally enervating. The drugs requested are almost always the *wrong* drugs.

I approach this work like a child to a bowl of boiled turnip. A strong sense of aversion. *This is work,* I tell myself, *not boiled turnips!* The aversion is, nonetheless, intensely felt. Existential nausea.

A person with fibromyalgia is requesting weak opiates for their pain. She has been taking them, I realize, for *years*. The effect will be disastrous. It always is.

A 22 year old requests a prescription for a selective serotonin reuptake inhibitor (SSRI). Started a month or two previously, she has missed her appointment for follow-up.

The parent of a child requests more methylphenidate. Then another child, then a 19-year-old student, then a 44-year-old father of two who is a solicitor, and I'm thinking *who is prescribing all these amphetamines?*

Then a request for benzodiazepines from an alcoholic.

More SSRIs.

Six requests for prescriptions for anti-diabetic medications which are unavailable now in the UK.

A lot of medication has become unavailable in the UK, since Brexit, since COVID, and I wonder, not for the first time, *why is no one talking about this?*

There are several prescription requests for anti-psychotics, for patients with emotionally unstable personality traits. One of them, I know, has just been released from prison. It is monstrous that she was sent there in the first place. Quetiapine 100 mg twice daily, enough to stun a cow. I swallow down hard on the injustice. I don't really have time to worry about that.

A run of prescription requests for eczema—emollients mainly, and I slide through these, slippery and friction free, like a child on a snow-slide, snagging only on some strong steroid cream requested for a 12 year old.

A request for dihydrocodeine from a 60-year-old cleaner with back pain. This time I make a note: *Call this one later.* The coward that inhabits me shrinks from the argument that I know this will cause.

My problem is that I haven't initiated any of these treatments. Each one fills me with doubt. It is as if the system itself generates them—and I haven't the time to chase each decision down to its origins. No one has that kind of time. But each drug issued represents a conversation that I am choosing not to have. Each represents the potential for harm. Time after time I move on to the next. A little chip chiselled from my integrity.

And I feel a kind of . . . moral nausea.

★   ★   ★

Caroline: The landscape of healthcare is continually evolving, expanding in scope, complexity, and reach. Medicine now responds not only to changing healthcare needs and demands but also to rapid technological advances, shifting delivery systems, and demographic transformations. In turn, healing and healthcare provision have become increasingly professionalized. Specialized. Institutionalized. Commercialized.[3]

The development of healthcare into a range of professionalized and specialized fields has been accompanied by a proliferation of medical specialties and sub-specialties. This transformation has included the emergence of new health-related professional roles. The physician—once equated with the very practice of medicine—now co-produces care within interdisciplinary teams. These teams bring together a broad range of professionals, each contributing distinct expertise and skills. The modern physician is no longer an autonomous healer, but one part of a larger collective. In this new role, physicians have taken on a wide array of novel tasks, while many traditional responsibilities have been shared or delegated to others.

At the same time, the healthcare system itself has grown into a dense network of institutions and regulatory structures—hospitals, clinics, insurers, pharmaceutical and biotech firms, government bodies, auditors, and knowledge institutions. These networks operate under varied logics—cost-efficiency, risk management, regulatory compliance—but are increasingly drawn together. Converging. Incentivized. Oriented toward realizing techno-scientific and economic potential. This transformation has come at a human cost. Several scholars argue that medicine is no longer guided by the integrity of care, but by the expanding demands of a system-world. A system that leaves little space for autonomy. Little space for moral integrity. The physician's integrity—that gravitational field pulling together diverse moral, professional, and knowledge-based commitments—is under stress. Pulled in multiple directions. Often contradictory. Responsibility for coordinating diagnostic and therapeutic paths has shifted from individuals to systems.

The result? Fragmentation. Of care. Of responsibility. Of responsiveness. As roles and routines evolve, the relational heritage of medicine—its emphasis on continuity, on personal care—has faded. In its place: Complexity. Specialization. Standardization. And with them, diluted accountability. This is what sociologist Ulrich Beck has called "organized irresponsibility"—a condition in which systemic complexity and diffused accountability make it increasingly difficult for individuals to act with moral clarity or take meaningful responsibility. The capacity for individual response—for response-ability—diminishes. It is displaced by the machinery of the healthcare system. The individual healer, once distinct, once whole, is now reconfigured through standardized competencies. Task sequences. Their lived experience—what they learn through care, through the burden and beauty of response—is now noise. Interference. Their suffering is not seen as knowledge. It is not even recognized. They themselves become diminished.

Diminished. Reduced. Alienated

Peter: I am! I feel it. I am *much* diminished.

What I actually *like*, in my job, is to engage with my patients. Person to person, face to face, standing with them, together, constructing with them a version of their personal situation, their personal struggle, in ways that make sense to both of us, help them to manage, and help us all, to live.

But I've no time for that right now, because right now I must process Test Results.

Mainly in the form of lists of numbers.

Long lists of numbers. The abnormal tests are typed in bold. Almost all the data sets, though, contain a number in bold.

My job is to ignore—almost—all of them. Almost all of them being clinically irrelevant.

Same problem as before though—I have ordered almost none of these tests. It's unclear often who has. The system, again. That stupid, blind system.

Haemoglobin a tiny bit . . . low. Ignore.

Platelets a bit high. Ignore.

A thousand cholesterol readings which are normal, or just a little high. Ignore.

Sodium low, potassium . . . high. Potassium is always a little high—it has to do with how long the sample has been left lying around before it was processed—unless it doesn't—in which case that can be *really* serious. Ignore anyway.

Calcium. Phosphorus. Vitamin B$_{12}$. Calcium again. Something called thyroglobulin antibodies—I don't altogether remember what they *do*—but they are OK, so I ignore them.

PSA 5.8

Prostate specific antigen. The clinical marker for prostate cancer in men.

Don't ignore.

(I shudder, sometimes, at the thought of how close I might have come to ignoring that. I comfort myself with the thought that all doctors think like this, that it's not just me. I worry, a lot, though, that it is, in fact, just me.)

Like many men of my generation, I worry a bit about my prostate. We're encouraged to. There is a general sense that we don't worry enough about our prostates—which have become metonymically representative of the whole of our mortal and moral selves. Men in the UK are encouraged to grow moustaches in November—we call it *Mo-vember*—to celebrate and promote this fact. A lot of moral anxiety gets focused on the walnut-sized gland at the base of our bladders, whether it contains cancer cells. I try not to worry about this kind of stuff—worry disables me—it incapacitates my creativity, prevents me from being the person that I wish to be, causing *me* suffering, so I fight against it. Nonetheless, like damp in an old house, prostate angst does seep through.

But still, don't put this work off. That *never* works.

I phone him. Let's call him Bill. He's 58. It sounds like he's at work. He sounds irritable, at least at first, when he picks up the phone.

"Yes?!"

"Hi. Bill. It's the doctor here."

"Oh." Now he sounds a little deflated. No one wants a call from their doctor, after all.

"It's about your blood test. Your prostate."

"My what?"

"Your *prostate!*"

These conversations can get very awkward, very quickly. There is the sound of muffled hands on the telephone, apologies to colleagues. He has moved into a private space.

"What about my *prostate*?" He sounds querulous. Like a child caught out, doing a bad thing, like he's been accused of filching a toffee.

"It's about a blood test. On your prostate. It's a little high."

"But I didn't want a blood test on my prostate! I didn't ask for that! Why did you do a blood test on my prostate?"

The truth is, I don't know. I try to buy time as I go through his medical record, trying to figure out *why did we do this blood test?* I'd be *furious* if I were him. Who ordered it? It's just not clear though. I deflect the question.

"There are a number of potential causes. Recent ejaculation! Infection! Cycling a lot!"

There is a silence on the line.

I teach young doctors, medical students, about communication skills. I *know* how badly this conversation is going. Don't judge me.

"Are you telling me that I've got cancer?!"

Maybe. Probably not. Who knows?

But now he's getting angry. People do get *very angry* about this kind of thing.

"No!" I say. "No! All we need to do is to repeat the test at this stage."

"When? When can I have it?"

"We need to wait. Perhaps in a month or two. I can book it in."

"Can't I have it done sooner? I want it done sooner! Can I *pay*? To get it done sooner?"

Medicine intrudes. I feel that myself. I fight against that in my own life. I have to. But it still gets in, and I am powerless to stop it. It can feel like an invasion: this alien, reductive force.

★   ★   ★

Caroline: Medicine intrudes. Breaks the person down into its component parts, as if it were these parts, and not the whole, that constituted the person.[4] As a strategy, it can be startlingly effective.

Modern medicine operates on the premise of strong causal relationships: between disease and suffering; injury and disability; medicine and health. Through empiricism and technology, it offers ways to mitigate these biological sources of anguish. Advanced technologies and specialized expertise allow for more precise identification of pathogens, dysfunctional organs, distorted tissues, dysregulated cells, and altered molecules. This approach has led to the classification of new and numerous diseases alongside the development of powerful interventions— vaccines, antibiotics, chemotherapeutics, immunomodulators.

In our time, the knowable—that which can be described in scientific terms—is often valued for what it enables. For what it allows us to act upon. This emphasis on action-oriented knowledge is a central feature of clinical spaces. In pursuit of clarity, certainty, and control, a focused and objective perspective has taken hold: what Michel Foucault famously termed the "clinical gaze." A disembodied gaze, sharpened by technologies of many kinds. It makes the body visible. Measurable. Calculable. Intelligible. And in doing so, it privileges these dimensions of the human.

For some, this approach is empowering. Biological data becomes a common language. It creates possibilities for shared understanding between patient and healer. At times, it works. At times, it works well. For others, it fails. For some, it becomes a source of pain.

The clinical gaze is reductive. It reduces people to data. Transforms them into problems to be solved. It is powerful but blind to the person behind the numbers. It cannot see the world through their eyes. Goals, hopes, dreams—the lived experience of suffering—fade from view.

The gaze is invasive. It leaves little room for secrets, for intimacy, for the private world. It makes the invisible visible. The unmeasurable measurable. But in doing so, it shifts uncertainty into concern. From "unknown unknowns" to "known unknowns." From silence to risk. It draws hard lines between normal and pathological. Between what is okay and what is not. Between what is good and what is bad.

The gaze is also alienating. It imposes its own logic. Driven by curiosity, ambition, and responsibility, it reconfigures the clinical space. Not as a place of listening, but of decoding. Not as a space of response, but of management. Those who are seen through it may feel detached from their own bodies. From their own meanings. Those wielding it may experience the same. In seeing, they may reduce. In reducing, they may intrude. And in intruding, they may harm. What once held the potential for encounter is thinned into a transaction. The relation frays—not through neglect, but through the very structure of how one comes to see, and be seen, in medicine.

The well become worried. The worried become patients. But some resist. They avoid medical advice. Refuse recommendations. Reject treatment plans. For them, the clinical gaze itself becomes a source of suffering.

Medicalization and Dehumanization

Peter: "A source of suffering."

These are not, however, the kinds of words that Big Tam uses.

He's more concise.

I try to avoid *his* gaze. His . . . glare—I skulk behind the desk at the reception so that he can't see me creeping back to my office. I took a break. Bad. A quick change of clothes was what I sought—I'm still sweaty after my cycle in. Perhaps even a quick coffee before I broach the rest of the day's work . . . but it is not to be, because Big Tam has already *seen* me.

"It's yous're the *effing* problem" are the *exact* words he uses. Tam is succinct. Direct. No scope for misunderstanding or ambiguity. He makes his point, clearly.

"Ah'm just after a wee bittie *compassion* here, just a wee bittie *kindness*, but it's aways the same—yous're all just *too busy*."

"If you'd just phone us, from 8 a.m., or better still, in advance, or alternatively, use our website."

Tam's a "walk-in." They mess the system up.

Anna, our receptionist, is trying to explain our appointment system. Which is so far beyond Tam's capacity to manage, we might as well have closed the doors and turned the lights off. Anna is trying her hardest to *de-escalate*. Heroically persevering with those scripts and conflict management techniques in which she has been trained. It's not working though.

"It's like yous cannae be *arsed*," says Tam, selecting from the milder of his repertoire of profanities. But Big Tam knows that if he goes all-in with the swearing he'll be thrown out, and *that* is something that he can't afford. He needs our help.

Tam, like many of the men around here, men of his generation, men of his limited repertoire of resource and opportunity, is addicted to heroin. He has run out of methadone, has been self-managing with alcohol and benzodiazepines. Now he is withdrawing, from *everything*.

Big Tam's not really that big. Actually, he's quite a shrivelled wee fellow—tremulous, hollow-cheeked, grey-skinned, life-altering crosses tattooed on his forehead, spittle and old food crusted in his beard. He's not stupid, although it would be easy to make that mistake. When sober, calm, in balance, there is a gentleness to him, a warmth, even. Ask him sometime about his big sister—how she cared for him as a troubled young man, kept him out of prison, kept him straight for a few years, before she died.

It's hard not to feel sorry for a luckless man like Big Tam.

At least in theory.

In practice, though, right now, he's gearing up for another round with our receptionist.

Anna's 19. Anna is kind and smart and capable and has a talent for this kind of work. I think sometimes that Anna probably has better communication skills than I do. More natural, at any rate.

"Sit down. Wait. I'll try," she says, but that's not good enough.

"I cannae *wait!*" yells Tam. "I've been waiting my whole *f★★king* life!"

At which point, too late perhaps, I step in, ask Tam to leave.

"No swearing, Tam!"

In our "clinical space" you're not allowed to use the "F" word. It crosses a line. A rather arbitrary line, but there you go—that's the nature of lines.

Big Tam storms out. Yelling at us words like *"Compassion!"* *"Care!"* and *"Kindness!"* as if they are weapons, which, in this context, they are.

Two young women with babies in buggies, just coming in for their appointments, watch, wide eyed, as the hurricane that is Big Tam blows by.

"Are you OK?" I ask Anna.

She rolls her eyes, smiles at me, says as if the question is stupid, "Of course I'm OK!"

I worry that this kind, capable woman is growing a shell. That hard, brittle surface that so many of us, to protect our softer parts, must grow.

I'm feeling less OK. I worry about moral injury. I return to my office, slump in my chair, resist the temptation to put my head in my hands.

The truth is, I quite like Big Tam. Part of me thinks he's right. He should be welcome here. He's just lost in the system. It can feel, at times, as if we all are.

★ ★ ★

Caroline: A man walks in, unwell, unruly, unscheduled. What he asks for may be difficult to deliver, but it is not difficult to understand. These are not extraordinary demands. And yet, spaces capable of receiving them—without filtering through systems of eligibility, triage, or suspicion—are increasingly rare. In late modernity, the clinical gaze has expanded, reaching far beyond the clinic to render life in terms of risk. But in the attempt to make suffering legible and manageable, something slips. What appears as disruption may be the clearest expression of need—misread not for its obscurity, but because it fails to conform to the forms of recognition the system has learned to accept.[5]

In late modernity, the clinical gaze has expanded, offering insights that reach far beyond the traditional boundaries of clinical spaces. Turned onto everyday life, it returns knowledge of risk—of exposures, habits, and conditions that quietly shape health long before illness appears. This reach is further stabilized by the rise of novel technologies that monitor and regulate these new dimensions of the medical. What once was confined to the clinic now follows people into their homes, workplaces, and daily choices, rendering ordinary life newly visible, measurable, and exposed. With the convergence of biological, informational, and communication technologies, entire ways of life are being reformed. Re-imagined. Through screening, prediction, and prevention. Under the premise that suffering can be precisely identified, understood, and addressed, both physical and mental selves are resolved into numbers. A myriad of data points become the foundation for clinical knowledge, for decisions and actions—actions no longer confined to disease, but extended to all aspects of health, the self, and everyday life.

This expansion has raised concerns. Concerns about overreach. What some have called "medicalization"—the reframing of intimate life as medical. Physical life. Mental life. Relational life. Social life. The costs of this reframing are real. Even when the benefits are too.

Overdiagnosis. Every medical label carries risk. Diagnostic labels can change lives. They can change how people see themselves—and how they are seen by others. They shape relationships. They shape identity. They can subtly, or dramatically, alter how people interpret their own existence. Overtreatment. Every intervention carries risk. Most interventions carry harm. When medical framings are applied where no pain or suffering was ever felt, the result can be deeply damaging.

In a world increasingly dominated by technologies, people—patients—can feel dehumanized. Still, it is hard to dissent. Hard to resist. People who hold values that diverge from the health norm may be seen as unintelligible. Unmanageable. They are labelled: "Non-compliant." "Difficult." These labels carry stigma. They carry moral weight. And sometimes, resistance itself is medicalized. Reframed as disorder. Addiction. Psychosis. Personality disorder. In these framings, agency dissolves. Responsibility is diminished. Resistance is no longer action. It becomes "behaviour." Not political. Not meaningful. Just noise. The creature pinned beneath the clinical gaze is lessened. Distorted. Dehumanized. As a moral agent. As a knower. And, finally, silenced.

This is not only a matter of individual harm—it is a relational act. The clinical gaze does more than observe; it positions. It produces asymmetries: Of knowledge, of authority, of moral worth. These are not just differences of degree, but of kind. To hold another in the clinical gaze is to see them through a lens that alters the terms of the encounter. What might have been a space of recognition or intimacy becomes structured by distance and control. And the cost is borne not only by the one who is seen. The one who sees—who is trained to interpret, to manage, to act—may also lose something essential: The capacity to encounter the other without reduction. Under the clinical gaze, both are at risk.

And yet, many still turn to medicine. They find solace in its frames. Not just for what it can do to the body, but for what it can offer the soul. For its promise of clarity. Its offer of recognition. Its ability to name and legitimize pain. People turn to medicine for explanation. For social validation. They ask it to translate suffering into something that makes sense. Often, the language of medicine is easier than the language of pain. Easier than the language of experience. A clear diagnosis carries weight. It brings status. It opens doors. The language of experience rarely does.

Medical Colonization and Social Control

Peter: I have a call to make. Something I'm dreading. I need to call a colleague about a child.

Call him Dale. He's ten and a half. His tragedy is greater than most children, but his story's not so unusual. It can feel sometimes as if there is a generation of children like him, marching lockstep with their cohort into a bleak and predictable future. Lock-down babies? I don't think it's so simple.

Dale's foster mother had called me earlier in the week. There's something not right about Dale; she wants him assessed. By a psychologist, perhaps. Or a child psychiatrist. She thinks he's ASD-ADHD.[6] Or possibly complex PTSD, given the horror of what this child has witnessed. It's as if he has a motor inside him. He never stops. He is destructive and oppositional. He doesn't sleep—he spends all night on a tablet computer, falls asleep at dawn, sleeps through the day. He hardly goes to school, and when he does, he can't be contained in a normal class—the other kids don't tolerate him, he bites and spits, they hit him back, so he spends his school days in the school "chill-out" space.

The foster mother, Mrs Mackenzie, as she austerely names herself, sounds a capable, smart woman. She is Dale's great-aunt. She says that she knew Dale would be a challenge when she took him on, but no one had warned her quite how much of a challenge. Social work had promised all kinds of support—he was acknowledged to be a vulnerable child—but nothing much happened, not really. Nothing that was helpful. She felt alone. All alone with Dale. She didn't know whether she was going to cope.

I remember meeting Dale, three years previously, with his birth mother. We had had a very similar conversation. She wanted him assessed for ASD-ADHD—the acronym, those disconnected letters—tripping from her tongue, as if they might be the perfect fit, the apt description for this child, her son, who was darting between the YouTube flicks on his tablet computer and the scales in the corner, which he would jump on, to hear it rattle, to see the dial spin round and around. I used to have children's toys in the corner of my clinical space, but children rarely play with them now. There seemed to be an invisible wall around Dale that I couldn't penetrate. He didn't seem able to hear me when I tried to talk to him—but I didn't try as hard as I might. To my shame, I felt no warmth for him, only hopelessness.

"I've tried my hardest, but nothing works," said his mother, but to my eye, she wasn't trying at all. She was ignoring him. I sensed, in my cold, hard heart, that she always had ignored him.

I referred Dale, back then, to be assessed by CAMHS.[7] I spoke with the school too—after too many missed calls—they were great, but they too had tried everything. I called social services—I was worried about Dale's mother—*her* lack of affect. I suspected that she was using benzodiazepines. I suspected that the mother's benzodiazepine use was half the problem.

Dale's mum died, of asphyxiation of vomit, from a drug overdose. Dale found her. That happened only a few months ago. I asked Mrs Mackenzie whether she thought that might be part of the problem? Grief? Trauma? But to my surprise, she thought not.

"But how can I tell?" she says. "I'm no psychologist. It's like there is a wall around him—nothing gets in, or out."

I made a promise to Mrs Mackenzie. I am careful about promises that I make—I am too much aware of the limitations of what the health services can offer, my own limitations too. I am wary of the harm that over-promising can do. But I said that I would try—to access some kind of help, for her, for Dale.

It takes forever to get through to the duty clinician at CAMHS. She is a little impatient with me.

"I can see that he was seen . . . two and half years ago. We thought he had ASD. Or perhaps FASD. He was started on melatonin. It seemed to help, with sleeping. I don't think they turned up for follow-up though."

"And so you just let him go?"

"Well, did *you* try to contact them?"

She sounds a little testy. I too have already raised my voice a little.

The tension between us goes like this:

We primary care doctors are overwhelmed by the demands of the parents of unhappy children. Their unhappiness is described by acronyms: ASD. ADD. ADHD. ODD. PTSD. FASD. Their parents, for whom I have nothing but sympathy, brandish these letters as weapons—demanding that their child be "assessed."

The specialist centres—staffed overwhelmingly by people who really *care*—are overwhelmed too. So overwhelmed, in fact, that a child referred routinely there might well *never* be seen. The parents say, "I'm watching my kid's childhood just . . . disappear."

Nothing is more pitiful than to hear that.

When the children *are* seen, they are assessed, and the assessments often run to many, many pages. Sometimes a prescription is suggested, as with Dale. Sometimes it is suggested that the parent attend a parenting class, but it seems they rarely attend.

Often our referrals are rejected. We are sent suggestions of a leaflet we may want to share with the parent or a website that they might wish to consult.

It feels like a fraud. Something has gone awry with childhood, in my country, at least.

We share some of this, over the phone, the clinician from CAMHS and I.

It must be unbearable for her, having these kinds of conversation with people like me.

Day after day, on the front line of the UK's child mental health crisis.

"I'm sorry that I have nothing more to offer for your patient," she says, and I appreciate her honesty.

"I know you're sorry. I'm sorry I raised my voice."

"It's OK. It's very frustrating. You could try writing to us and saying that he's at risk of killing himself. He might get seen then?"

"That would be a lie though. I can't do that."

"No. I understand that."

"We're powerless, aren't we?"

"Totally. Powerless."

We share a moment, she and I. It's comforting, in a way, to acknowledge this. It makes us feel a little better.

Poor Dale. Blameless. Trapped by circumstance. A nexus of invented medical labels, intractable social despair, institutional powerlessness. It's as if the child himself had never existed.

These feelings we have, of regret, will, of course, make no difference to *him*.

★   ★   ★

Caroline: A child's intimate experience. All that nuance, complexity, hope, despair. Anatomized and objectivized by a range of labels—labels which define entities that are, at best, unstable in their nature and their implications. And, at worst, social inventions—contingent on accidents of history and culture.[8]

It can seem as if the human, existential world—that world of contingency and suffering—is constantly intruded upon. Encroached by a world of systems, processes, discourses, and conversations which may seem "science-y" but are no more usefully descriptive of the world than that which they seek to replace.

But why? Who benefits?

The social significance of the clinical space far exceeds its ostensible purpose. Perhaps that has always been the case. Healing practices have long been a part of how humans imagine themselves into being. Modern medicine is no exception. It is productive—not only in the tangible sense, in the production of health and cure—but also in how it generates identities, societal norms, and social expectations. Gradually, medical authority has expanded into political and social domains. And, in this context, the clinical gaze is no longer limited to physicians and healthcare professionals. The clinical gaze has become a way of understanding the world and acting within it.

A lens through which the modern world is viewed. A grammar through which political ideas are conceived. A prism through which pasts are re-interpreted and futures re-imagined.

The tools of medicine—its ways of seeing, measuring, interpreting, and understanding—serve not only to improve individual lives but to shape society as a whole. Medicine has become a means not only of offering assistance but of interpreting needs—relationally, politically. It functions as a mode of moral action, shaping how worth, vulnerability, and responsibility are assigned. Its measures and metrics do not merely track health—they signify something more: Development, progress, value. And when these standards are not met, they do not register only absence or lack. They mark failure. Social. Political. Even moral failure.

Medicine's expansion beyond its traditional borders is marked by paradoxes. First, the tension between liberty and control, expansion and restriction, freedom and constraint. Second, the quest to diminish disease has coincided with a proliferation of diagnoses, complaints, and despair. How did a project aimed at emancipation come to carry so many new burdens? What kinds of suffering are alleviated—and what kinds are created—when medicine extends its reach?

Medical expansion was once legitimized by its power to heal. Increasingly, however, it reflects broader power dynamics. The mechanisms that drive this expansion reveal how deeply medicine is entangled with the society in which it is embedded—how its logic and reach are shaped by technoscientific promises, commercial interests, and regulatory demands. In Latour's terms, medicine is no longer a purely clinical actor, but a hybrid—part scientific, part social, part political—produced and sustained through dense networks of institutions, tools, expectations, and imaginaries.

Medicine has expanded under the premise of liberation from suffering and premature death. Yet it now operates within the confines of a new biosocial order—one that is both expansive and limiting. Medicine has become part of the apparatus of social control. This influence is not enforced through overt authority or coercion, but through what Michel Foucault calls subjectification—the subtle internalization of norms, practices, and discourses that is productive of subjectivity itself—how one comes to understand health, normalcy, and identity. Within this framework, health is no longer just a condition to be maintained or restored; it becomes a moral imperative, a measure of responsibility, even a form of virtue. To be healthy is to be good. To fall outside this norm is not only to be at risk but to risk becoming unintelligible. And with this there is now a moral, even legal, expectation of participation. Both patient and practitioner engage actively in the medical encounter. They participate in the development of technologies, practices, and frameworks. The clinical encounter increasingly takes the form of a transaction—an exchange of services, rights, data, or recognition—with each party accountable to systems that measure value, compliance, and outcome. Citizens, too, have become invested—often as demanding of medical validation and recognition as clinicians themselves.

This shift toward the clinical space as a site of transaction carries profound consequences. Patient "autonomy," expressed through requests, demands, and choices, leaves little space for deep listening or ethical response. The danger is that something fragile, ambiguous, unspoken goes unnoticed. The other's need is often not declared in advance; it does not arrive in the form of an articulated request. It is sensed, felt, suffered. In this light, the philosopher Emmanuel Levinas speaks of the call of the other—not a statement or question, but an interruption. An ethical demand that arises before it can be named. When the encounter is shaped by what is already requested, already chosen, already medicalized, it is this call that is too often drowned out. The space between caller and responder narrows. The relationship becomes constrained, reduced, and shallow.

Medicine, once confined to specific places and times, now saturates life. From individual experience to social participation, everyday life is organized around the pursuit of health outcomes. Illness and suffering are no longer only biological; they are cultural, narrative, interpretive. But medicalization obscures this interplay. It reduces identity and context to data, pathology, and intervention. In the world made visible through the clinical gaze, there is little room for the social, the relational, the particular. There is no language to describe it. No frame to hold it. No way to know it. And in this, failure is inevitable.

Suffering, in its raw and unprocessed form, often presents as existential. Loneliness. Fear of death. Despair. Disappointment. When such suffering is reframed as biomedical, the possibility of existential remedy is lost. Human solutions to human problems move out of reach. When pain is relational or political, medical framings may not just miss the mark—they may obscure the very solutions rooted in relationship and social context. Relational solutions to relational problems. Social solutions to social problems. Political solutions to political problems. All moved out of sight.

As medicine has extended itself into political, social, and private spheres, healthcare professionals increasingly find themselves constrained by the very frameworks they once helped to build. They, too, have become bound. Fixed in and by the clinical gaze. Their work and identities reduced. Dehumanized. Intruded upon. Colonized. The knowledge that arises from the lived experience of caregiving, from the weight of responsibility, from the act of being responsive, and at times from the pain of being unable to respond is dismissed as noise, as interference. Their own complex, personal kinds of suffering are veiled. Silenced. And with that, their capacity for moral engagement is diminished.

The Gap, the Challenge, and the Possibility

Peter: And I do find myself so bound: Fixed and constrained by this *clinical gaze*: By expectations which seem unconnected to any relationship I may seek with my patient, and my patient with me.

What might it mean to free myself? And if I did, would I still be doing medicine at all?

My first real appointment of the day, my first *face to face*, is with Alasdair.

Alasdair will help cheer me up, though that's not really his job.

Alasdair is like an old hawthorn, shaped by the west wind: As wise as one, with something of the posture too, leaning, stooped, battling into an unknown future.

45

Alasdair, help me to express what it is that I'm struggling to say here.

Alasdair carries the burden of a gradually progressive illness. A disaster, perhaps, life-limiting, for a man in his 40s or 50s; more manageable for a man in his late 80s.

I see him every month, for about ten minutes. He requires a painful, somewhat technical procedure—an injection with a large-bore needle into the abdomen. Now that I think about this, I think that it is something that could easily be carried out by a nurse. I enjoy his company too much to suggest that, though.

I suspect, with little evidence, that he doesn't always trust people easily. Certainly he's no fool. He brings me the kit for the injection, together with a print-out of very detailed instructions for its administration. He brings me a fresh copy every time. I could feel insulted by this, I guess, but it feels to me to be a considerate act—he doesn't just take it for granted that I have the (fairly meagre) technical skill to carry out the (simple enough) procedure—even though I have done it now 30 or 40 times. It feels like kindness on his part. And I still follow his instructions meticulously, as I prepare his injection. Perhaps I just have no pride.

Over the years we have maintained a wide-ranging conversation. We covered poetry (he's a Gael, a fan of Norman Macaig and Sorley Maclean, Gaelic poetry generally); a little politics (despairing, head-shaking); neuroscience; languages; business management; family; the pleasure and pain of raising children to be adults; America; Ireland; music, particularly folk music, particularly the joy of unskilled musicians jamming together in small spaces whilst drinking alcohol; Middle Eastern history; and hill walking. Ten minutes a month, over three or four years. That's more than enough for a proper chat.

"How was your Christmas holiday, Doctor?"

"Beautiful. Hung out with friends. Swam in the sea."

"Weather?"

"Chilly. Clear."

"Where were you?"

"Near Arisaig."

"Ah . . . beautiful. Views over to the Isle of Rhum. And Skye!"

"The Cuillin Hills."

"On a clear day."

"There was snow."

"I've never walked there myself."

I mix the drug with the solvent in the barrel of the syringe, affix the needle, swirl it a little more to ensure all the particles are dissolved. I wash my hands again, I change my gloves.

I think of the piercing white of the Cuillin ridge of Skye, covered as it rarely is in snow, the beauty of that serrated edge. I have the flicker of a memory of a weekend spent with a friend, almost ten years ago, when we walked from one end of the ridge to the other, slept overnight on its rocky crest, witnessed the sun set beyond the peaks of St Kilda, the morning's weather already blowing in.

I don't need to say anything, Alasdair's already making his way to the couch.

"How was your holiday?"

"Good!" He hesitates. "My brother's getting home."

Alasdair's brother has been in a nursing home after an incapacitating stroke. His recovery has been slow, he's been too long cradled in the love of his family, only now, months later, taking baby steps to independence.

"My sister-in-law thinks that I have been rather too bossy."

I raise an eyebrow. I swab the area where the injection will go. We alternate sides. I can never remember which side to go. Alasdair keeps me straight. Points his finger at the right place.

"I'm too full of suggestions for his recovery. Over-organizing. I tried to arrange rehab and physio. She took me aside."

"What did she say?"

"She reminded me of how angry I was, when the family kept on interfering, telling me what to do, when my first wife died."

I hadn't known that he had had a first wife. I had assumed him eternally, happily married to one. *Why?*

I lift a fold of skin, find the tissue plane, plunge the needle, inject the solvent.

"The funny thing is, I had no memory of being angry at all with them, not then. I don't remember being upset. I don't remember that at all."

"When was that?"

"Thirty . . . something . . . years ago."

A little younger than I am, now, I think, doing that thing that humans do, connecting his story to my own. I withdraw the needle, press some cotton to the tiny wound, which bleeds profusely.

"What happened to her?"

"She had a brain tumour. For the first couple of years after, I just wanted to die. Then I felt just . . . sad."

I put some tape on the cotton wool, turn away. I take off my gloves, wash my hands again.

For two years, I just wanted to die.

In another, imagined world, one which has never been, and will never be, I am he. I see things from the perspective of the younger man, and I think, *Will I ever overcome this sadness? Will I ever want to be alive again? Will I ever stop missing her? Will there ever be pleasure or joy in my world?*

"Then I recovered. I began to feel some happiness again."

I sit. He sits.

I'm aware that I have tears. I'm aware that he does, too. There is a little silence: That moment when a trapeze reaches the top of its swing, before it falls; the moment between one breath, and another, before there is movement again.

"I think about her now though, more and more. These last couple of years. Mainly at night."

Generally, at this point, I will make another appointment for Alasdair. In a month.

I fiddle with the computer, scroll through some dates.

"I find myself . . . filled with regrets."

In sympathy, I find myself drowning in regret. My own.

I swallow hard. I leave off fiddling with the computer. Listen again.

"For the little things, the big things, the stupid things I did."

"All those stupid things," I say, commiserating.

"She loved her work. She worked in the police. She was good at it. Our kids were at a difficult stage. I insisted she give up her job. I really, really, upset her. But I was earning enough for both of us. I thought she would be more useful at home."

For a moment, he looks emptied out, almost translucent. That stupid, despotic, younger man; the bereaved widower in his early middle age, longing for death; the old man, haunted, but wise, as a hawthorn tree shaped by the wind—these three men and their ghosts, sitting there, shaking their heads, filled with regret.

I shake my own head, say "So stupid," thinking mainly of myself, of all those stupid things, all the regrets.

"I'll see you in a month?" I print out a sticky for his next appointment. He is already writing it, the date, the time, in pencil, in his diary, in a meticulous hand. We stand. I touch him on the shoulder. We both shake our heads, laugh a little.

What on earth was that about?

"Goodbye."

"Goodbye."

★　★　★

Caroline: When suffering is misinterpreted or silenced failure becomes inevitable—failures of knowing, failures of moral engagement. It cannot be otherwise. Yet from such failures, new possibilities may emerge.[9]

In the clinical space, patient and practitioner are entangled—not only in asymmetrical differences but also within an intimate community. Subjugated by the same structural, cultural, and narrative forces, they are bound in and by the same gaze. They participate, together, in the dialogue of care. This creates a shared landscape of experience—a terrain marked by common struggles against some of the root causes of contemporary suffering. And in shared suffering, a different kind of understanding is possible. Through attentive listening—to self, to other, and to the wider structures that shape them—one may access a privileged kind of knowledge: rooted in the clinical space, yet straining beyond it. In this mutual space, voices of pain may rise to speak not only of injury, disease, and disability but of fragmentation, reduction, alienation, dehumanization, and colonization. Medical understanding may begin to shift. No longer confined to anatomies and diseases, it may expand to include human realities. Humane realities. Societal realities. These are forms of knowing that not only shape care but also illuminate its place within a fractured and fragile social world.

Such experiences are not peripheral. They are central features of the human condition in late modernity. Actively listening to this pain—bearing witness to it, amplifying voices bringing it forth—may open a way forward: A path that is at once personal, relational, and social. A path that offers not just knowledge but a reweaving of meaning, integrity, and relation.

The question "How to respond to the suffering other?" becomes, first and foremost, the question. But the answer can never be fixed or final. It must be rearticulated and reenacted—within each encounter, within each structure, within each moment where suffering rises to speech.

We listen then—attentively—not only to the individual voice but to the relational spaces and social worlds that voice carries with it. Only by hearing suffering afresh—each time as if for the first time—can we properly answer it. Only in this can there be response-ability.

We're All in This Together

Peter: Today, right now, I'm pondering all of this.

All these contradictions and tensions. How they imbue our practice.

Such as: There is a world, inside of myself, where I live. I imagine that you have one too. And then there is the one outside, in which we are embedded—which we know imperfectly but which sustains us. There is an inner world and an outer world, and there is this gap between them. And there is the question of how these two worlds and their different substances can possibly connect. How do they find a common language?

I know that these aren't new worries, but they seem very real, to me, today.

Or, this—what was the *medical* part of that consultation that I had yesterday with Alasdair—that gentle man, who still seems to haunt me? His ghosts, and what these ghosts evoked in me? All those regrets, come home again? Or the expensive drug that I administered, which helps keep his death, for a while, at bay? Which mattered more, and how?

And, I think, not for the first time, that the thing that connects all of this, somehow, and binds it all together, is the thing we call *empathy,* but I don't really understand what that thing is, what that mystery word really means.

The ostensible purpose of medicine is to mitigate suffering. But the scope of objective medical knowledge ends where the subject begins. There is a gap between, a gap of knowing—an epistemic gap. It is as if these domains of knowledge existed in different universes, ruled by a different logic, with different grammars, and different words.

The language of science and medicine can describe, eloquently, the cause, mechanism, and effect of, say, a pain, but nothing of what that pain is *like*, what it might feel like, and what it might mean to its subject. Only the subject can do that.

Medicine can't fulfil its ostensible purpose without adopting both perspectives. Standing firstly *with* the subject, with his unique knowledge, trying as if to see the world through *his* eyes . . . whilst, simultaneously, standing as an outsider, objectively, seeing the subject *as* an object of knowledge.

There is a contradiction here, but it runs deep—it's woven into the fabric of how things *are*. The presence of such a contradiction can be terrifying. It can seem to threaten the very basis of how we understand the world. But seeing where our understanding fails is the precondition for change. We can't progress without first knowing ourselves to be wrong.

This is the contradictory space: The knowledge space in which the healer must operate. This is the domain of our special skill. Understanding the tensions and contradictions inherent there, its potential for healing, for suffering, and for truth, is our challenge.

This is our super-power, our challenge, and our commitment. To develop skills of listening, the skills of curiosity and humility. To be the agent that can transcend this gap, the shaman that crosses these domains. The ones that have the courage to speak—that can give voice to suffering. That is *our* responsibility.

But I wasn't thinking that yesterday, not then. Then, I was far too busy. I had too much to do.

Then, yesterday, I just closed the door behind him. I sat for a moment. I gathered myself.

Thought: *Next.*

Notes

1 This voice draws on conceptual foundations indicated in the endnotes, including key traditions in the sociology of late modernity, medical sociology, anthropology, science and technology studies, and feminist theory.
2 This section draws on key works in medical anthropology and sociology and the sociology of late modernity, framing the clinic not only as a site of diagnosis and intervention but also as a reflection of broader social currents.

- Arthur Kleinman, in *Patients and healers in the context of culture* (1980) and *The illness narratives* (1988), situates the clinical space within cultural systems and moral economies of healing.
- Deborah Lupton in *Medicine as culture: Illness, disease and the body* (3rd ed., 2012), explores how medicine reflects and shapes contemporary cultural norms.
- Ulrich Beck in *Risk society: Towards a new modernity* (1992) and Zygmunt Bauman in *Liquid modernity* (2000) theorize late modernity as an era defined by fluid identities, systemic risks, and a moral imperative to self-manage.
- Anthony Giddens in *The consequences of modernity* (1990) highlights how reflexivity and institutional destabilization structure everyday life.
- Hartmut Rosa in *Social acceleration: A new theory of modernity* (2013) offers a lens on how institutional and technological tempos compress the experience of time.

Together, these works illuminate how clinical encounters become ethical and existential sites in which identity, responsibility, and vulnerability are negotiated.

3 This section builds on foundational works that examine the transformation of medicine from an autonomous profession into a complex, institutionalized field shaped by broader systemic forces.

- Eliot Freidson, in *Profession of medicine: A study of the sociology of applied knowledge* (1970), analyzes how medicine established itself as a powerful profession through claims to specialized knowledge and self-regulation.
- Paul Starr, in *The social transformation of American medicine* (1982), traces how professional autonomy was gradually undermined by the bureaucratization and commercialization of healthcare, leading to medicine's increasing entanglement with institutional and market logics.
- Ulrich Beck, *Risk society: Towards a new modernity* (1992), introduces the concept of organized irresponsibility, describing how distributed systems obscure individual agency and moral clarity, creating a landscape in which responsibility is felt everywhere and nowhere at once.
- Sheila Jasanoff, in *Dreamscapes of modernity: Sociotechnical imaginaries and the fabrication of power* (2015, with Sang-Hyun Kim), offers the concept of sociotechnical imaginaries—shared visions of progress that fuse science, policy, and institutional design—highlighting how healthcare systems increasingly orient themselves toward technoscientific futures rather than relational or ethical coherence.

Together, these thinkers illuminate the growing tensions between care, coordination, and control in contemporary healthcare—revealing how institutional complexity can dilute moral agency and obscure the embodied, relational knowledge once central to clinical practice.

4 This section builds on foundational critiques of biomedicine's objectifying tendencies, exploring how medical knowledge reshapes perception, erases subjective experience, and risks alienating both patient and practitioner.

- Michel Foucault, in *The birth of the clinic* (1973), introduces the concept of the clinical gaze: a disembodied, objectifying mode of knowing that renders the body visible, knowable, and governable—while effacing the patient as subject.
- Georges Canguilhem, in *On the normal and the pathological* (1978), critiques medicine's tendency to enforce rigid distinctions between normal and pathological, masking the lived ambiguity of health and illness.
- Drew Leder, in *The absent body* (1990), explores how medical practice displaces the lived body, leaving the subject estranged from their own experience.
- David Armstrong, in *Political anatomy of the body: Medical knowledge in Britain in the twentieth century* (1983), examines how modern medicine produces new ways of seeing, classifying, and acting on the body as a political and institutional object.

Together, these thinkers illuminate how the gaze of medicine—however clinically effective—can be deeply reductive. It privileges what is measurable, calculable, and visible, often at the cost of intimacy, personhood, and relational care. The result is a practice that can heal the body, but sometimes only by silencing the voice of the one who suffers.

5   This section draws on key thinkers who have shaped understandings of medical authority—its expansion, its promises, and its ethical costs.

- Peter Conrad, in *The medicalization of society: On the transformation of human conditions into treatable disorders* (2007) and earlier works with Joseph Schneider, *Deviance and medicalization: From badness to sickness* (1980), trace how medicine increasingly defines and governs areas of life previously seen as moral, social, or personal.
- David Armstrong, in *Political anatomy of the body: Medical knowledge in Britain in the twentieth century* (1983) and *The rise of surveillance medicine* (1995), examines how the clinical gaze has shifted from diagnosing disease to managing risk—reaching into everyday life through preventative regimes and health surveillance.
- Nikolas Rose, in *The politics of life itself: Biomedicine, power, and subjectivity in the twenty-first century* (2007), explores how biomedical technologies have reshaped identity, morality, and responsibility, giving rise to new norms of health citizenship and self-regulation.

Countering these expansive logics, several thinkers emphasize the moral asymmetries and relational wounds created by these developments:

- Jonathan Katz, in *The silent world of doctor and patient* (1984), critiques how institutionalized medicine renders patients passive, voiceless, and morally judged—especially when they resist dominant framings.
- Havi Carel, in *Illness: The cry of the flesh* (2014), offers a phenomenological account of illness that centres lived experience, vulnerability, and the limits of medical knowledge.
- Annemarie Mol, in *The logic of care: Health and the problem of patient choice* (2008), proposes an alternative to autonomy-based models of healthcare grounded in attentiveness, adaptation, and relational responsibility.

These thinkers help illuminate how the clinical gaze, though often well intentioned, can disqualify alternative forms of knowing, restructure agency, and create hierarchies of intelligibility. In doing so, it shapes not only how people are treated but also how they are understood—and how they come to understand themselves.

6   ASD = Autism spectrum disorder; ADHD = attention deficit hyperactivity disorder. These acronyms are often combined together in common parlance. A person is often described not in terms of *having* these, but *being* these. See also FASD = fetal alcohol spectrum disorder; PTSD = post-traumatic stress disorder; ODD = oppositional defiant disorder.

7   CAMHS = Child and Adolescent Mental Health Services.

8   This section draws mostly on theoretical work that explores how medicine has come to govern not only health but also identity, citizenship, and moral life. It situates medicine as a key site of biopolitical power—shaping what it means to live well, suffer properly, and be intelligible.

- Michel Foucault, in *The birth of the clinic* (1973), inaugurated a critical tradition that sees the clinical gaze not simply as a medical perspective, but as a mechanism of power that objectifies, classifies, and governs through visibility.

- Thomas Lemke, in *Biopolitics: An advanced introduction* (2011), expands on this foundation, showing how modern governance works through life itself—regulating populations through norms, statistical expectations, and internalized responsibility.

- Bruno Latour, in *We have never been modern* (1993), shows how science—including medicine—operates through hybrids that blur the line between nature and society, revealing its deep entanglement with social, political, and institutional forces.

- Ian Hacking, in *The social construction of what?* (1999) articulates how categories of personhood, particularly in the medical and psychological domains, are not fixed but looping kinds—they interact with those they describe and reshape behaviour, policy, and subjectivity.

- David B. Morris, in *The culture of pain* (1991) and *Illness and culture in the postmodern age* (1998), explores how suffering is culturally shaped and narratively mediated.

- Roberto Esposito, in *Terms of the political: Community, immunity, biopolitics* (2012), explores the paradoxes at the heart of biopolitical projects: How efforts to protect life often generate exclusion, vulnerability, or new forms of domination.

- Emmanuel Levinas, in *Totality and infinity* (1961), offers a different emphasis—one not focused on systems of classification or control, but on the ethical demand that emerges from the vulnerability of the other.

Together, these thinkers make visible how medicine, far from being a neutral or purely curative practice, has become one of the central infrastructures of late modern governance. It defines health not only as a biological state but as a moral ideal, extending into every aspect of personal, relational, and political life—and often foreclosing the possibility of existential, relational, or social remedies for suffering.

9 This reflection draws on traditions in narrative medicine, feminist theory, and care ethics that understand listening as both a form of knowledge and a moral act.

- Rita Charon, in *Narrative medicine: Honoring the stories of illness* (2006), frames listening as a clinical practice that opens space for meaning, dignity, and transformation.

- Arthur Frank, in *The wounded storyteller: Body, illness, and ethics* (1995), shows how stories of illness resist reduction and reclaim agency, and how the listener becomes a co-witness to suffering.

- Donna Haraway, in *Staying with the trouble: Making kin in the Chthulucene* (2016) and earlier work on situated knowledge and entangled lives, offers the notion of response-ability—a form of attentiveness rooted not in control, but in the capacity to stay with complexity, discomfort, and the demands of relation.

Together, these thinkers affirm that to listen is to respond and that response-ability begins not with solving, but with being present—ethically, emotionally, and intellectually—to what suffering asks.

4

When Death Comes to Work

Margot de Rijke

Some days, like today, the ER was a death sentence.

Stefan Delaro had pancreatic cancer. The tumour lit up on the screen like a large white mass lodged in between his small intestine and his stomach. Even without the biopsy, it was unmistakable.

Yesterday, he had been a history teacher at a nearby high school who took his dog out for hour-long walks, watched every single one of his teenage boys' basketball matches, and shared a bottle of red wine with his wife on Saturdays.

Today, he was dying.

Beatrice had been annoyed when she first spoke to him.

"I've been feeling a little . . . off," he said. "Like something isn't right."

She was pushing his abdomen, trying to provoke that feeling of unease he described. "Any pain? Nausea? Are your stools any different from normal?"

He'd shook his head, and she had decided he wasn't worth her time. She would simply check his labs and send him home with a referral to an endoscopy within a few weeks. Nothing to be afraid of, but he was in the right age to have his colon checked anyway.

DOI: 10.1201/9781003593294-4

Then he'd added, "I've lost some weight." *8 kilos over the past month.*

She'd looked at him. A slender man, too thin to willingly be losing weight.

So she had ordered a CT scan, because suddenly she, too, had a feeling that something wasn't right. And now she had the answer. This man was dying, quicker than anyone would have thought when he walked into the ER a few hours earlier.

Beatrice sighed and squared her shoulders. Delivering bad news was not something she enjoyed, but it was part of the job. Better get it over with.

But before she could find her way up to the surgical ward on the third floor where he had been given a bed, she was interrupted by her pager. A quick call told her a 17 year old had an appendix that was about to burst and he needed surgery right away. Stefan Delaro's death message would have to wait.

Secretly she was glad.

★   ★   ★

The appy was followed by an incarcerated hernia and then a perforated ulcer. Beatrice had been in the operating room long into the night, and when she could finally sit down in the thankfully deserted office she shared with Lilith, Stefan Delaro was not on the forefront of her mind. But when she logged on to her computer to gauge the situation down in the ER, it was his records that sprung up on her screen.

Beatrice always prioritized informing the patient about their diagnosis, even when it was a less-than-pleasant message. But it was late and he was probably sleeping, and there were other patients waiting for her. This conversation required time. And his wife. Both of which were lacking at the moment.

It would have to be tomorrow, when Delaro was awake and Beatrice's shift had ended. One of the other doctors would have to do it.

She downed a bottle of lukewarm water, did a few stretches, and returned to the ER, ready for whatever problems were waiting for her there.

Beatrice had two hours left of her shift when a nurse called from the surgical ward. Delaro's blood pressure was plummeting and he was talking gibberish. *Sepsis.*

"Give him fluids and start antibiotics. I'm on my way."

When she came storming into his low-lit room a few minutes later, there were three nurses standing around his bed. He was hooked to two IVs, and one of the nurses was putting ECG stickers on his chest. There was also a urine catheter sticking out from the standard white hospital underpants that hadn't been there before. The man himself was looking distraught, suddenly much older than he'd looked a few hours earlier, and was obviously scared of everything that was happening.

"How is he?" Beatrice asked the room at large.

"Tachycardic."

She nodded. "BP?" "Stable. For now," the nurse added grimly, staring intently at the monitor.

Beatrice looked at her patient. He was looking back, eyes wide and his glasses askew. "Wh-what is, uh. . . . Where am I?" he asked, voice quivering. "S-Sarah." *His wife.*

One of the nurses grabbed his hand and gave it a squeeze. "You're in the hospital." She spoke in a clear tone that made Beatrice suspect that she might have told him that several times already. "You have an infection that we need to treat."

The nurse then turned to look at Beatrice, the doctor in the room, to see if there was anything else that should be added. Beatrice swallowed. Too many things were happening at the same time. It was late and he was severely ill and his wife wasn't here. Also completely delirious. Now was not the time to inform him that the infection was caused by a large tumour that would soon kill him.

"Give him morphine if he needs it and put up another bag of fluids when this one is done," she said. "Call me if his vitals change."

Then she disappeared, unable to stay any longer. There wasn't really anything she could do anyway, other than wait for the fluids and antibiotics to do their work. In the meantime, all he needed was a cold cloth to his fore-head and continuous monitoring, both of which were outside of Beatrice's job description.

She returned to the ER once more.

The next time the nurse called her up to the ward, Delaro's vitals had dropped even further, his breath now stilted and his legs swelling. Beatrice stood in the room while he died, silently watching while a nurse held his hand.

5

Medicine: We Make It; It Makes Us

Eivind Alexander Valestrand and J. Donald Boudreau

Do I contradict myself?
Very well then. . . . I contradict myself;
I am large. . . . I contain multitudes.

"Song of Myself" (Whitman, 1891–1892)

Imagine a skilled actor on stage. What the audience sees is a polished performance—confident, deliberate, and carefully executed. The protagonist springs to life through compelling gestures, poignant facial expressions, and convincing tone. However, behind the costumes and a proficient delivery of scripted lines there are numerous layers; some are conscious and intentionally concealed, others are unconscious but discoverable, and some are non-conscious or inaccessible. Each performance is given shape by prior interpretations, influenced by cultural traditions, and informed by evolving socio-material contexts. The actor's portrayal of a specific character arises from years of training in public spaces as well as personal struggles that have played out in private or secret spaces. Every rendition arises from a plethora of experiences—harsh critique, constructive feedback, silence, recognition, validation, epiphanies. These result in the accretion of numerous emotions, including some that lead to self-doubt, self-esteem, or self-delusion.

This chapter seeks to explore the multitudes, as evoked in the epigraph to this chapter, within a doctor's identity. It asks the following questions: What is a professional identity? How does this identity evolve over time? How is it shaped by a substrate of personal values, societal expectations, and professional

DOI: 10.1201/9781003593294-5

experiences? How do unseen drives and impulses, both internal and external, affect the kind of person they become, what and who they come to care about, and how they provide care? To understand a doctor's identity, we must attempt to look beyond what is illuminated by the spotlight focused on centre stage and consider the forces operating behind the curtains. Unseen layers of effort contribute to singular portrayals and, perhaps, unique identities.

We have chosen to use the actor as a metaphor with which to initiate the conversation. We acknowledge its limitations. Every metaphor opens doors to understanding while closing others. They create opportunities and impose new constraints. We toyed with alternative metaphors; for example: (i) The iceberg—we appreciated its ability to shine a light on layers that are deeply submerged; (ii) a storage cabinet—it would allow for the examination of contents in different drawers—some fully open, some ajar, and others shut tight; (iii) lenses—they might open up a discussion of entities and experiences that can reveal constituent parts but that also have the potential to distort, that can lead to formation and also to deformation. We landed on the actor (and acting) metaphor, but we accept that it can easily be problematized. Two obvious drawbacks are the suggestion that the portrayal of a role or character can be transient or temporary and that the portrayal may not be syntonic with the actor's authentic self—if such a thing exists. We believe that a professional identity is much less evanescent than the rendition of a particular role; it is more permanent than that. A professional identity "gets under the skin" in a more commanding and indelible fashion. Despite such limitations, we believe that the actor metaphor has value. Also, a dramaturgical approach is grounded in the literature; it summons the concepts of "presentation of self in everyday life" and "image management" as described by Erving Goffman (Goffman, 1959).

In the public eye, doctors step into the role of the professional—the white coat, stethoscope draped around the neck, the decisive presence offering lucid and logical diagnoses and treatment plans. However, as implied earlier, underlying this performance lies something far more intricate: A reigning and powerful medical culture, a lifetime of experiential learning with skills acquisition and the building of competence and confidence—but also injury, at times leading to vulnerability and at other times to resilience. Just as an actor's portrayal is shaped by context, emotions, and personal history, so too do power structures, discourse, beliefs, doubts, and the weight of responsibility influence how doctors practise medicine and navigate their place in the world (Helmich et al., 2017). Within unseen dimensions there may be contradictions and complexities. These shape every professional interaction and every decision.

What Is Identity?

None enter medical school as blank slates (tabula rasa). We bring with us lived experiences that shape who we are, the values and beliefs we hold, and the reasons we feel called upon to study medicine (Sternszus et al., 2024). These form the foundation of a doctor's identity—an expression that captures how we understand ourselves, the world, and our place within the world and how we believe others perceive us. This identity influences how doctors engage with their patients, their profession, and the larger society.

Doctors bring their personhood to the practice of medicine. It affects how they perceive health, illness, suffering, and healing. For example, a doctor whose family were refugees and had a strong family bond while striving economically may value compassion and see medicine as a means to social justice, advocating for underserved populations. Another doctor, shaped by his father surviving a lung cancer due to successful surgery and chemotherapy chosen to fit his tumour's characteristics, might focus on technical precision. These perspectives are not in opposition, but rather different expressions of how one's worldview is deeply embedded in personal and professional identities.

Moreover, worldviews sensitize doctors to the experiences of others. A doctor who witnessed their grandmother endure the sharp, debilitating pain of trigeminal neuralgia—a condition characterized by intense facial pain—might draw on this personal experience to better understand and support a patient with chronic pain. Conversely, a doctor whose worldview is shaped by a strong belief in self-reliance and resilience may view pain management differently, emphasizing coping strategies and functional recovery over emotional validation. In this way, a similar clinical encounter can unfold in markedly different ways, shaped by the doctor's underlying values and assumptions.

This worldview-driven identity interacts with and is shaped by the world itself. Doctors operate within systems—hospitals, societies, cultures—that impose expectations, values, and pressures on them. These forces can both reinforce and challenge individual approaches to care. A doctor practising in an overburdened emergency department may begin their career by valuing thorough, patient-centred discussions, but gradually adapt to an environment where rapid decision making is paramount. Over time, they may find themselves adjusting their approach—not out of personal conviction, but because institutional structures reward efficiency over deliberation.

As a consequence, the 40-year-old man with chest pain in the emergency room may be discharged in the middle of the night when lab tests and heart monitoring are normal, leaving the doctor to overlook the anxiety, existential suffering, and suicidal thoughts that manifested as chest pains. In such cases, the system does not necessarily strip doctors of their compassion, but it conditions them to prioritize what is measurable and immediate over what is complex and human. This ongoing negotiation between personal convictions and systemic constraints illustrates how a doctor's identity represents a dynamic interplay between internal values and external influences.

Identity is not a fixed script; it evolves as doctors grow, learn, and adapt to the challenges they face and the settings in which they perform. Yet, at its core, it represents how a doctor sees and engages with the world, and it powerfully impacts every aspect of their practice, their relationships, and their sense of purpose.

Struggling to Form a Professional Identity

Our personal identity, largely shaped during childhood and adolescence, plays a critical role in the kind of doctor we eventually become. Who we are before medical school significantly influences the identity we develop as physicians.

In one author's case (EAV), much of his identity as a future doctor was shaped by experiences as a patient. He writes:

As a child, I suffered from severe asthma, which resulted in frequent hospitalizations until I was about four years old. Throughout my early school years, I had to take medication several times a day, sit farther away from bonfires than my classmates, and I sometimes struggled to breathe during sports. Though my asthma improved as a teenager, another challenge soon followed. Between the ages of 13 and 18, I endured chronic vomiting, often many times a day, as doctors tried and failed to find a clear explanation. Eventually, I was diagnosed with a degenerative neural disorder that affected my stomach, preventing food and stomach juices from moving through my digestive tract. I was surgically treated by removing my stomach, gradually improved, and became able to return to school and social activities.

These experiences profoundly formed the basis of the person I was when I entered medical school. Forming an identity as a physician was no gentle process. The most difficult part of my medical training wasn't memorizing facts or understanding theories; that simply required time, effort, and discipline. The real challenge lay in the identity shift that was happening within me.

Stepping into the role of a doctor was an emotional battle that meant letting go of my patient self. I had to confront deep-seated parts of myself, parts that had grown accustomed to seeing the world from the perspective of vulnerability and illness. Reimagining myself as someone who could heal, who others would look to for strength, was daunting. It forced me to question how I fit into the world, not as someone being cared for, but as someone responsible for the care of others.

In the case of the other author (JDB), his childhood upbringing was marked by the influence, and at times the intrusion, of religion. He writes:

My parents were observant Roman Catholics, and although it was implicit and assumed rather than overtly stated, they endorsed a philosophy closely associated with the "theology of liberation" movement. The latter's critical and emancipatory view of the world order permeated my everyday life, even in prayers, leaving an indelible footprint on my worldview. This background was a preparation and a natural fit for medicine. Aspects of my personal identity nurtured by this philosophy, notably altruism, service, and justice, were concordant with values that medical doctors have often professed. The alignment (sometimes perceived as much as real) facilitated my entry and adaptation to the medical education trajectory. It also compelled me, shortly after graduation, to sign up for a two-year engagement with a volunteer association in Latin America, a Canadian equivalent of the Peace Corps or Médecins sans frontières.

The professional journey was not always smooth sailing. My religious background was the main source of core values that conflicted head-on with certain medical practices considered standard and routine in the communities where I lived. Assisting in first-trimester abortions was the prime example. This widely accepted feature of the medical mandate required me to examine deeply how I might find a professional niche where I would be able to don the habit of the medical doctor, without rancour and a feeling of self-betrayal.

These experiences are far from unique. Although much of who they are can be *consonant* with the professional role they are trying to fill, medical students or doctors occasionally encounter what can be called an identity *dissonance*—a tension between their personal and professional identities (Costello, 2006). Such dissonance is not inherently negative; it can serve as a powerful catalyst for growth. Rather than resulting in the proto-physician feeling as an "imposter within," it can prompt self-discovery and permit previously underdeveloped aspects of their identity to emerge and become integrated with professional values.

Identity dissonance can be emotionally complex, especially if embracing a professional identity requires letting go of deeply rooted aspects of oneself. For instance, seeing oneself primarily as a patient or having a strong religious identity can necessitate a re-evaluation of self and a softening of these roles to accommodate the evolving professional self. A process that involves relinquishing core aspects of personal identity, such as changing how to view one's past, one's friends or family, can be painful. Still, there is an expectation of a reward in the end that makes the road worth the travel.

For others, the tension between personal and professional identities is not merely a challenge—it costs them more than it gives. They may find it difficult to reconcile the professional identity expected of them with deeply held personal beliefs or values. A doctor who entered medicine with a profound commitment to holistic healing may struggle in a medical culture that emphasizes diagnosis and intervention over human connection. Rather than feeling like they are growing into their professional role, they may experience a sense of loss—as if the deeper, humanistic motivations that led them to medicine are being eroded. This struggle can manifest as moral distress, disengagement, compassion fatigue, or even a crisis of meaning, where the practice of medicine feels less like a calling and more like an institution that demands conformity at the expense of individuality.

Grappling with identity dissonance can ultimately lead to four possible outcomes, which may be distinct, blended, or alternating over time. A doctor may leave the medical field entirely; resign themselves to living with conflicting identities, increasing the risk of emotional exhaustion and burnout; resist change while striving to reshape the professional culture; or find a way to integrate personal and professional identity. For those who can interweave their personal and professional selves, the result is often a richer, more authentic sense of self. For instance, developing an identity as a doctor does not mean abandoning empathy or the understanding of suffering. Rather, it may allow past experiences as a patient or caregiver to be transformed into compassionate and effective care for others and thereby also demonstrate that the individual physician can compensate for dehumanizing tendencies in "the system" of healthcare institutions. In embracing the discomfort of change, individuals may not only uncover a clearer sense of who they are but also gain insight into who they aspire to become.

Relational Capacity

There are existential aspects of being alive that all humans share and can relate to—such as searching for a greater meaning in life, experiencing suffering, and being mortal. Doctors are by the very nature of their work exposed to these existential realities, which profoundly influence how a person understands themselves and their role in the world. The ability to recognize shared human experiences—such as fear, hope, vulnerability, and resilience—can help doctors relate deeply to those in their care. It fosters empathy, allowing doctors to see their patients not just as cases to be solved but as fellow human beings navigating the complexities of life. In turn, these interactions may shape the doctor's identity, reinforcing the understanding that medicine is not just about curing illness but that the good clinician should feel concern for, be attentive to needs of, and, perhaps most importantly, be curious about the patient and interested in their well-being.

Strengthening doctors' relational capacity—their ability to connect deeply with patients—can serve as a powerful tool for advancing health equity. By recognizing universal dimensions of suffering, vulnerability, and resilience, doctors can bridge gaps that cultural, racial, or socioeconomic differences might otherwise create. For this to happen, medical education needs to tend to the subjectiveness of their students, recognizing them as unique persons that can learn to use their experiences, emotions, and vulnerability to connect deeper with the patient to understand their tailored needs. If future doctors can do this, we can gradually change the medical culture into one where the personhood of the patient is considered as exciting and important as their disease and its characteristics. Such a relational approach encourages physicians to see patients from diverse backgrounds not only by their unique challenges but also as individuals navigating the same existential questions that bind all of humanity.

When a strong relational capacity is part of their identity, doctors can move beyond implicit biases or surface-level cultural competence, fostering genuine curiosity and empathy. It prompts a deeper exploration of how systemic inequities and social determinants of health shape the experiences of minority patients, while also allowing doctors to reflect on their own assumptions and perspectives. Such a reflective process can enrich both the doctor's identity and the therapeutic relationship, creating a space where vulnerable groups feel seen, heard, and valued.

Through connecting with patients, the doctor's self-understanding can become intertwined with the broader existential questions of life: Who am

I as a healer? What is my role in the suffering of others? How do I navigate my own emotions while caring for those in need? These questions are not only intellectual. They are deeply felt, a changing force shaping how doctors perceive themselves, their profession, and their relationships with others.

The Boundaries of the Profession

Our personal journeys have given us our ways of seeing the world—and a clearer understanding of the role we wanted to take in it. We have realized that there is no single, prescribed way of being a doctor. The profession needs to offer room for individuality, allowing physicians to grow into the role while holding on to the core of who they are. This is essential. Becoming a doctor, developing a doctor's identity, cannot only be about becoming part of a profession, socializing into thinking, acting, and feeling like a stereotypic doctor. It needs to be about developing oneself as a doctor *within* the profession.

While there must be room for this individuality in how medicine is practised, the profession is also defined by clear standards and expectations that set boundaries for acceptable behaviour. Not everything is permissible. But what should guide us in determining acceptable physician behaviour? How can we establish a framework that serves as both a boundary and a space for personal expression?

The answer may lie in the virtues of medicine. Beyond scientific knowledge and technical skills, the practice of medicine requires doctors to embody qualities that reflect a commitment to the well-being of their patients. A doctor must interpret clinical realities with curiosity about what an illness means for the individual, recognize the importance of demonstrating compassion for the patient, respect their autonomy, communicate truthfully, exhibit courage in the face of uncertainty, and uphold fairness in treating all patients equitably. In essence, doctors are called to embody moral excellence.

In their book *The Virtues of Medicine*, Thomasma and Pellegrino identify trust, compassion, prudence, justice, courage, temperance, and effacement of self-interest as essential virtues in medicine (Thomasma & Pellegrino, 1993). These virtues provide a moral compass, guiding doctors to navigate the complexities of their work with integrity and humanity. Trust can foster meaningful relationships with patients, compassion can lessen suffering, and courage enables doctors to make difficult decisions in uncertain or challenging circumstances. Temperance, meanwhile, guards against over-reach, and the effacement of self-interest reminds doctors that their duty is first and foremost to the patient. Together, these virtues establish the ethical boundaries of the profession while leaving room for the individuality necessary to practise medicine authentically.

Still, missteps are inevitable. When the expectations for doctors are so high and the pressures of the workplace so intense, the boundaries of the profession are often tested. Moments of moral failure or professional misjudgement may arise—not necessarily due to a lack of virtue, but because of the immense complexity of modern medicine and the human limitations of every doctor.

Virtues are learned, understood, and embodied through role modelling and reflection and by asking difficult, unsettling questions in the medical world in which the value of each virtue is made immanent in the actions of those acting there. Excursions to the edges of the profession's boundaries can provide profound opportunities for growth. The ability to reflect on mistakes is essential for navigating the complexities of medicine, but it also requires embracing imperfection without succumbing to harsh self-judgement. For some doctors, their sense of self is so tightly intertwined with their professional role that missteps can feel deeply threatening. In contrast, those with a more balanced identity—perhaps encompassing facets beyond their work as doctors—may find it easier to withstand and learn from such moments of failure.

One of the authors of this chapter recently encountered a pair of frustrated parents whose family life was unravelling due to their son's severe behavioural challenges. They felt ignored and abandoned by the healthcare system, despite a record that showed prudent adherence to clinical guidelines. The child had benefited from a thorough diagnostic process. Standard treatment protocols were initiated. A request for medical approval of absences was denied because the rationale was deemed clinically inappropriate. Everything had been handled correctly—by the book. Yet from the parents' perspective, they had not been helped. During the meeting, the parents requested a sleeping medication that was not specifically indicated. The technically correct approach, according to guidelines, would have been to ask them to carefully chart the child's sleeping pattern, offer guidance on how to deal with sleep hygiene, and withhold medication, at least for the time being. But instead, the medication was prescribed—not as a primary solution, but as part of an effort to rebuild trust and foster a therapeutic alliance. It seemed that compassion demanded that the doctor break the rule. Most of the meeting was spent listening to their frustrations, validating their struggles, and acknowledging their resilience in caring for their son under such difficult circumstances. This approach was about more than following guidelines—it was about ensuring the family felt that someone had seen, heard, and supported them in a system they believed was working against them. While imperfect by the standards of strict protocol, the co-enactment of compassion and courage reflected the doctor's identity drawing towards the deeper moral calling of medicine: To care not just for diseases and patient categories but also for the persons who endure health problems.

Permitting virtues to be a deeper guide for what is appropriate physician behaviour provides an opening for compassionate rule breaking. Such transgression of rules and guidelines are, of course, open to criticism and not risk free. Thus, it demands courage of the physician—a core virtue of medicine.

Conclusion: The Doctor as a Human Being

A doctor's identity is vast, multifaceted, and often shaped by what happens both in and out of the spotlight. The visible performance—the professional attire, the clinical composure, the calm demeanour—gives us a sense of who the doctor is. Yet these outward characteristics represent only a fraction of the true self that exists behind the scenes.

As doctors move through their careers, they wrestle with the weight of their profession, continually negotiating between the personal and the professional, being a healer for others while tending to their own needs. Identity is not static; it shifts and evolves through training, practice, and the ever-present demands of care. Behind the curtain, a doctor carries their personal values, emotional complexities, and moral dilemmas—factors that shape their performance by impacting their decisions, empathy, and capacity to connect with others.

The tension between the external image of the doctor and the internal experience is an ongoing one, often marked by contradictions. Doctors may at times be seen as detached or unemotional, but within them may lie a well of compassion, resilience, and vulnerability that too often is suppressed by convention or fear. In moments of crisis or self-reflection, their professional and personal selves become more visible, revealing the depth of their humanity.

Ultimately, understanding a doctor's identity requires seeing them not just as medical professionals, but as individuals deeply intertwined with their work and their world. Their identity is an expression of how they understand themselves, medicine, and their place within medicine and how they believe others perceive them.

References

Costello, C.Y. (2006). *Professional identity crisis.* Vanderbilt University Press.

Goffman, E. (1959). *The presentation of self in everyday life.* Bantam Doubleday Publishing Group.

Helmich, E., Yeh, H. M., Kalet, A., & Al-Eraky, M. (2017). Becoming a doctor in different cultures: Toward a cross-cultural approach to supporting professional identity formation in medicine. *Academic Medicine, 92*(1), 58–62.

Sternszus, R., Steinert, Y., Razack, S., Boudreau, J. D., Snell, L., & Cruess, R. L. (2024). Being, becoming, and belonging: Reconceptualizing professional identity formation in medicine. *Frontiers in Medicine, 11,* 1438082.

Thomasma, D. C., & Pellegrino, E. D. (1993). *The virtues in medical practice.* Oxford University Press.

Whitman, W. (1891–1892). Song of myself. In E. Folsom & K. M. Price (Eds.), *Leaves of grass* (pp. 29–79). Walt Whitman Archive. http://whitmanarchive.org/published/LG/1891/poems/27

6

Levels of Experience

Lara Kesseler and Peter Dorward

This chapter is an email correspondence between two general practitioners, a younger one (Lara) and an older one (Peter) who know each other well, reflecting on how they experience and exist in the world of doctors and patients.

Dear Peter,

I have been mulling over what we talked about and paying closer attention to my recent consultations. I feel I have always been aware of how factors like fatigue, time of day, and my general mood change a consultation. I have been less aware, however, of what you called the "doctor's suffering." It made me think of a patient I saw a while ago. She was in her 50s and had a diagnosis of CFS, chronic fatigue syndrome. She had checked her own blood pressure at home and realized this was low, which it had always been, but she now felt this was abnormal considering she was middle-aged, overweight, and postmenopausal. The symptoms she experienced from her chronic fatigue syndrome had recently flared but were, in essence, unchanged from the pattern it had always followed. However, she was now wondering if her low blood pressure could explain her symptoms and, if her blood pressure was linked to her symptoms, then surely we could treat it and she could move on with her life feeling better than she did before?

I thought it was unlikely such a link existed, but I still felt obliged to do at least a few blood tests and to examine her.

It was during our follow-up consultation that a strong sense of inadequacy bubbled up in me.

DOI: 10.1201/9781003593294-6

Because I didn't have a simple explanation for her symptoms, I couldn't give her a treatment that would make it "all better." I find it hard, this expectation, or maybe perceived expectation, to "fix" things. I realize there are very few things in medicine you can truly cure, and I don't generally struggle with this. It is, however, the symptoms I can't clearly explain which I find much harder to deal with, partly because it leaves me with a feeling that maybe it is my lack of knowledge or experience that is the problem, that there should be something I can say or do to help. So, in this case, I made it sound like a positive thing: All her blood tests were normal, this was good because at least nothing was seriously wrong. I acknowledged how she felt split between relief and disappointment and then I hung up the phone. Feeling like I didn't do a good enough job, feeling inadequate.

Best wishes,
Lara

* * *

Dear Lara,

These stories are always interesting, in a painful kind of way.

Doctor suffering is real—I've experienced it myself, more times than I would like to say, and supervising trainees, watching them consult, listening to their stories, about how they get things right, and get things wrong, and how they react—I know that it's not just me. The suffering comes in many flavours—shame, fear of criticism, the moral distress of "letting someone down," the fear of letting yourself down, emotional overload, powerlessness. I could go on. My minimal claim is this: That clinician suffering, in its many forms, influences the outcome of our clinical encounters. And we never talk about it.

Why would the case that you describe cause you suffering though?

There is a lot of hostility in the world, directed toward doctors trying to manage the kind of case that you describe here. Chronic fatigue syndrome. Fibromyalgia. Menopause. Each, to different extents, gendered forms of suffering. No one claims that we manage these problems well. There are plenty of voices out there making that very clear. Go on the web, social media, old-style newspapers, Google reviews for your practice—you get the sense that some people out there hate us. The emotional stakes feel high before we even start.

It seems to me that there are (at least) two quite distinct ways of approaching this case. In the first, you might think, people alive in the world have always contained within them a deep, dark pool of undifferentiated suffering. Whether the total amount is about the same or whether it gets better or worse, I don't know. I suspect, without evidence, that it's about the same. But the way that suffering is perceived and expressed in the world depends on culture. The language of suffering changes across countries and down through history. That changeability doesn't make the nature of the suffering less real or less important. But if this is the case, your job is to have the skill to understand this person in all their uniqueness. To understand the language in which suffering speaks and is performed through this individual. It's a challenge. But it offers hope that you can find mitigation that you and your patient will make sense of.

Alternatively, you might go with the majority doctor view and think nah. . . . Because Addison's disease isn't just a story. Hypothyroidism, oestrogen deficiency, type II diabetes, undifferentiated connective tissue disease, and leukaemia aren't artefacts of culture, and neither is coeliac disease, for that matter. And if you miss any of these infinite possibilities, the patient will, rightly, be annoyed, and you will feel terrible. We have all suffered in this way, too. We prioritize illness that we see as, somehow, real. We talk about diagnoses of exclusion. Narrative doesn't even begin to do that. We are frightened of blame and guilt; the consequent suffering. But there are risks associated with this approach too. How do we begin our search? And, more importantly, where do we end? And can it be right to investigate our patients because we are frightened?

Does it happen sometimes, that in trying to find that rarest of fish, we let the whole catch go?

I find myself caught in this dilemma all the time. I would like to say that it gets easier with age, but I'm not sure that it does.

In practice, we run both approaches simultaneously. Either we perform as materialist doctors, steeped in technological medicine, with a bit of skill in empathy and understanding too, or we are skilled holistic healers of suffering, reaching across diverse cultural traditions, yet with knowledge and expertise in the physical body—how it suffers, how fast, or slowly, it dies.

We ride both horses—on a good day skipping between them, galloping along, adept; on a bad day, falling in the dust.

What do you think? Is this a dilemma that you recognize? How do you see the way forward?

With best wishes,
Peter

★   ★   ★

Dear Peter

You have given me a lot to think about. At the same time some of it provokes immediate ideas and opinions that then on second thought might be too black and white. It made me realize how two seemingly similar cases can have a completely different outcome. I have been trying to analyse why certain consultations take the direction they do, or as you say, how my suffering determines the outcome.

In the first example I gave you, I felt empathy and therefore I wanted to help and felt inadequate when I couldn't. A very similar case, however, provoked completely different feelings and with this the outcome was completely different. This woman was in her 40s with a busy life and young kids. She had been struggling with fatigue and had seen the GP about this. Shortly after this, she had a dizzy spell and sustained a head injury that resulted in her having post-concussion symptoms for a longer-than-average time. When I spoke to her, she was very much in a mindset where she wanted answers and solutions—she wanted to know why she had become dizzy; she did not want to hear that symptoms of a head injury can remain for months (her CT scan was normal); and, above all, she was angry, she was suffering, and she wanted it to end. Rationally, I know that these emotions come from a place of frustration, maybe even fear. Emotionally though, it makes me feel anger because of the combative way she approached me and frustration that she can't accept (yet, at least) that there is no magic cure to solve her symptoms. I still find it hard to separate her emotions from mine, to realize that her anger affects me but not to blame her for the feeling that it evokes in me. These are my anger and my frustration. Needless to say, we did not leave that consultation on a good note. I think she felt unheard by me, and I was irritated because I felt she asked of me something I could not give, and she did it in a way that made me feel she was demanding it.

You mentioned that you think the amount of suffering in the world is unchanged but that it looks different depending on where in the world you are. I sometimes think that we in the Western world no longer expect certain forms of suffering. I know this a bold statement to make, I have not thought it through in detail, and I might completely change my mind on it again. That being said, sometimes I feel that with increasing technology in healthcare we act as if being healthy in our younger years has become a right, that every problem has a clear answer and a cure or at least a good treatment. That there is no tolerance when this is inevitably revealed as an illusion and things turn out differently than expected.

This patient for me represented this—the idea that I can do a test, give her some medication, and can tell her exactly when she will be healthy again. I realize I am projecting these ideas on to her and I might be entirely wrong, but it is in essence why a patient like this makes me frustrated. I feel that she has unreasonable expectations which I cannot meet, and I resent her for asking this of me.

Writing it down in this way makes me realize how much is left unsaid in this consultation, how much I am interpreting her silences, her tone of voice and weaving this into my own narrative. Maybe they are true, or maybe they are a complete fabrication of my own mind. Processing it this way at least helps me understand myself a little bit better and perhaps it will help me to respond with a little more kindness next time.

Best wishes,
Lara

★ ★ ★

Dear Lara,

I like where you are taking this!

I'd like to take it a little further.

I think, though, that to do that, we'll need to take a bit of a dive into what it is we mean when we talk about suffering.

I'd like to suggest, for the sake of our conversation, a really broad, really capacious account of what we mean by the word. I think that when I talk about "suffering," what I intend is any kind of threat, real or imagined, to the integrity or existence of our self. I know that that raises a bunch of other questions—questions going off in all sorts of directions. What do you mean by "a self"? What about pain? How sentient does a thing have to be to count as a "self"? But notwithstanding a thousand possible worthwhile debates and diversions about the details, I still think that this definition provides a kind of flexibility and suppleness that is useful. It allows the word to do the work that is demanded of it—allows for its sheer range of application—from the worst possible kind of suffering, to something quite trivial, transient, and apparently unimportant. The whole range of our experience, as suffering beings.

I think that that is necessary. If we accept two premises—that any medical consultation contains within it the presence of at least two suffering entities—the patient, and the doctor—and that doctor suffering is therefore a potentially determinant factor in any medical consultation—then we have the potential scenario of a person, a patient, who is suffering in the worst possible way, being ignored, or forgotten, by a doctor, because that doctor is hungry. Or angry, or running late. Or tired. You can imagine the outcome of one person's suffering depending on another's. You can just imagine this scenario arising. Quite often, actually.

Or conversely, a patient, careless with another's feelings, says or does something that so impairs the doctor that he ceases to function—to his detriment, and the detriment of the next or subsequent patient upon whom that suffering is so commonly dumped. You will have had, no doubt, the experience of being shouted at, or sworn at, threatened, or just used. You know what that does to us.

Are you familiar with these scenarios? I am. They fill me with fear—their own, unique kind of suffering.

So I think that even trivial suffering can matter—our own, everyday trivia, can matter in its own, non-trivial way!

Suffering occurs in its context though. What Edvin would call our "existential anatomy." That is, this predicament that we all have in common, which we all face, as a consequence of our natures. Being mortal. Being alone. Being obliged to make meaning and purpose in a universe that, in itself, lacks these things.

So suffering is immanent, everywhere and always, stitched into the fabric that composes us.

This is part of the challenge and pleasure of our work. The manner by which these huge philosophical concerns intrude, constantly, unexpectedly, into our day to day, in ways that can be in turn bleak and pitiful, awe inspiring, irritating, hilariously funny. It is quite unpredictable.

You say that "I sometimes think that we in the Western world no longer expect certain forms of suffering" and "[it seems that] every problem [must have] a clear answer and a cure or at least a good treatment." I think you're putting your finger on something important. These thoughts stir something uneasy in me.

When a patient confronts us with whatever it is that ails them, something is engaged in us. You describe it well: "I find it hard . . . to separate her emotions from mine, to realize that her anger affects me." From the first moment of the encounter, one way or another, we're networked in. We begin to feel, just a little, how this person's life—in all its complexity, ambiguity, and pain—might be to them.

But something about the tradition of our training funnels us back towards a kind of bio-technological simplicity. The desire to convert complex, situated suffering into an objective problem that can be defined and fixed. You know the cliché—"to a man with a hammer, every problem is a nail." By bending complex, messy situations into solvable problems, we reify them. That is, we reduce them to formulas, turn them into things: things that can be counted, assessed, processed, acted upon. We disentangle ourselves from the complexity of our patients' suffering, make something objective, simple, and well known from the subjective and uniquely complex reality of their experience.

That's amazing, in some senses. After all, so much of what is good in medicine comes from its technical, scientific power. The bright, revealing light of its rationalism. Its power to know. Let's jettison all these old-style guys with their fusty three-piece suits and beards, crouched, muttering to themselves by the sick bed, a finger resting theatrically on a pulse! Why not? We're all better off in the world of things that can be fixed. Try breaking your leg or having a baby. You'll be pleased with the technology then!

But even then, even in the simplest, most transactional case, it can feel as if something has been taken away. In the shadow of the cure there remains, unevaded, the reality of our situation. There is no cure, only amelioration. However we ignore them, our deaths still walk with us, silent companions. To deny their presence is to deny our own selves. Our cures can then become a form of deceit.

What do you think?
P

★ ★ ★

Dear Peter,

I remember my brother once saying he wasn't ready to sign up as an organ donor because he wasn't ready to contemplate the possibility of his own death. This seemed strange to me at the time—but maybe that is because as healthcare professionals we are confronted with the inevitability of death so often. I agree with what you say about there not being a cure, only amelioration. But how often do we put it in such frank terms when talking to patients? I feel that often we skirt around the subject until we have no choice but to name it because death suddenly has come too close to comfortably ignore its existence. Still, even though we are guilty of this, it would always amaze me, especially when working with the elderly, how little people talk (and maybe think) about it. Even people who, by modern standards, are considered old.

I remember on a night shift being asked to speak to the son of a woman who was 97. She was admitted with an infection and antibiotics had proved to be ineffective. Really, she was dying. The dayshift medical team, after long conversations with the family, had decided to stop life-prolonging treatment. I was asked to speak to the son, because he wanted us to start subcutaneous fluids in order to give his mother, as he put it, "a chance." By the time I saw her she was not responding to my voice, her hands and feet were cold, and her breathing had started to change. I discussed with the son why I did not want to start her on fluids, but could see that he did not agree with me. He seemed to be clinging onto the hope she would get better. He kept telling me how healthy she had been until this current illness.

Two hours later she died. When this happened, the son seemed to change. It was like a burden had been lifted from his shoulders. It seemed that suddenly he could accept the fact of his mother's death and be at peace with it. I remember finding it strange that someone would be so unwilling to let go while she had reached such remarkable old age. Later, I wondered whether the fact that he had advocated for her allowed him to feel that everything had been tried—and that, in turn, gave him what *he* needed—to accept the inevitable.

It all makes me reflect on the question of whether those patients—and their families—that are more accepting of the fact that you can't live forever are the ones that have a more peaceful death. But then again, perhaps trying everything that modern medicine might have to offer is just what some people need to help them on that path to acceptance. But then, where do you draw the line? And to what extent does or should the patient and family have a say in this?

What do you think?

Best wishes,
Lara

★   ★   ★

Dear Lara,

I think that we are asking questions that are important and useful. And I think—I know—for sure, that it's better to ask these questions than not. And I think that often we doctors don't or can't have these kinds of conversations because we lack the time, space, or vocabulary to do so and that failure is to our own and to everyone's detriment.

We don't talk or think enough about our own and our loved ones' ends. That's my view. Our reluctance to have these conversations with our patients, and our perception that our patients are reluctant to discuss these things with us, are an extension of this, our deep reticence, when confronting the hard truths of our situation. So, I have this sense that I think you may share, that it would be in some way "better" for your brother if he were to set aside a little time, from time to time, to think, to make the necessary accommodation with his situation. But he doesn't really want to, at least not yet. He is, in his words, "not ready."

So you ask the bigger question—how passive should we be in the face of our patients' "not readiness"—their existential reticence? How respectful should we be of our patients' right not to know? Especially when we sense that, deeper down, knowledge is what they really want or need?

I'm sure you will be familiar with the situation of the bereaved, demented person who asks continually, every day, where their deceased loved one is. (I can picture such a patient now—the look of abandonment, the utter distress on her face, imploring, "where is my son?" The son who died, years ago.) None of us should brutalize others with the truth, wanted, needed, or not. That seems clear enough.

But on the other hand, the patient who is prepared—who knows what she needs to know—who has done the necessary emotional "ground work"— just seems to do so much better! And I do think that we can help with that.

I have such a patient, right at the moment. Relatively young, she had some routine blood tests that showed a not very spectacular abnormality of her liver function. She is quite asymptomatic. An ultrasound, then CT, showed a dilatation of the biliary tree, and a provisional diagnosis was made of cholangiocarcinoma. She was told that the tumour was unlikely to be treatable but was nonetheless offered a more elaborate series of investigations to establish and refine the diagnosis and potential options. After the initial shock of the diagnosis, she came to me to discuss her situation. She couldn't understand how she could be so ill, yet feel so well. I adopted the metaphor of the "plateau." She is in the "plateau" stage of her illness—with the implication that this would be temporary, that sooner or later, she would come off the "plateau." The metaphor landed, as they sometimes do, and she adopted it. "I like it," she said, "up here on the plateau. The view's good. You can see a long way."

We hit it off, she and I. I enjoy her visits. She asks me from time to time about what it might be like, when her time comes to come down off her plateau—what that process will be like. We have quite detailed conversations about what it is like to die. As if I could possibly know. She isn't interested in medical treatment that might be futile, and most of all, she isn't interested in anything that will upset her peace of mind—this strange end-of-everything tranquillity that she seems to have found, on her plateau. So she declines most offers of investigation or treatment. I'm comfortable with this. I'm comparatively realistic about the limits of medical technology, and so quite sanguine, most of the time, when patients decline it. I would go so far as to say that I feel better after our regular conversations. We meet once a month. It seems like an unequivocally useful investment of time, to act as this admirable woman's guide, helping her to find her way around on her plateau and, when the time comes, to help her to find the best, the safest route back down.

But I have a suspicion that my comfort with her decision, and my willingness to engage with her in her reflections about her mortality, is feeding, and sustaining her decision. To a certain extent, I might be colluding with her. Certainly, her family, from time to time, look askance. Sometimes her husband attends her appointments with her and weeps silently as she makes her humorous hill-walking-as-metaphor-for-death observations, which he only half understands. Recently, a family member asked her to ask me to reverse her DNAR order (do not actively resuscitate), which she had previously asked for. They felt that that was premature—and perhaps they are right. Who can know?

The thing is, there can be no such thing as a "neutral" guide. Like it or not, if I try to engage with my patient, properly, as a fellow human being, then my ego is in that space too, with all that that entails: All of my own half-acknowledged prejudices, needs, fears. We're all players, all of us who are involved. I don't think that we would want it otherwise.

In our society, time, culture, we privilege this idea of "autonomy." Rightly, I think. I wouldn't have it any other way! The "first amongst equals" of ethical precepts. But it sometimes feels that we misunderstand what "autonomy" is or what it entails. It can seem sometimes as if we imagine autonomy to be an isolated, unconnected thing—this thing that must be "respected." I think that autonomy, if it is to mean anything, must be understood as relational in its nature—that relationality is built into the concept—there can be no autonomous subjects without other autonomous subjects, and it is the interaction between them that gives the concept its philosophical teeth. So the idea of "respect" for autonomy might be useful as a working rule of thumb—especially when there is disparity of power between the subjects involved—especially when there is such an historical background of paternalism, patriarchy, injustice. It seems then that most of this "respecting" is quite properly going to be going in only one direction. But this idea of "respect" shouldn't obscure the underlying reality. Autonomy is always relational. The process, to be meaningful, works both ways. It's always an interaction, and that interaction is the space where medicine, understanding, and healing happen.

So too with suffering. Suffering is the flip side of autonomy. It may be contingently helpful to see it as an objective thing that needs to be identified, quantified, analysed, fixed—but that will only ever take us so far. The reality of human suffering is that it, too, is relational in its nature. By its nature, it is always experienced in the context of others who are, or have, or will suffer.

How might all of this be useful, or relevant?

Actually, I don't think that's too hard to answer.

I do this exercise sometimes with junior doctors or students who are sitting in with me, watching me consult.

It's very simple.

I ask them, before we begin, to make a list of all of the people they can think of whose influence might be affecting the journey and outcome of the consultation. After the patient has left, we make a list.

It always seems to start with, "Well, obviously, there's the patient."

"Well, obviously."

Then, sometimes with a little coaxing, the student will acknowledge me. My suffering.

"True, you did seem a little tired—a little distracted at times."

"Anyone else?"

Silence.

"Did you notice how the patient came alive when you talked? I asked you to ask her this or that, and you did, and she really came alive."

The student often seems a little surprised that they—with all their doubts and anxieties, fear of failure, enthusiasm, callowness, youth—will have added anything that matters—but so often they do.

"Anyone else?"

It turns out that others were mentioned in the consultation. A parent or a child. Another doctor, or a nurse, or a therapist. A person recently born. Or recently dead. Or a writer, TV personality, influencer, campaigner. Sometimes God gets a mention, often ancestors.

Often it can seem that there is an entire cast of characters, some real, some fictional, alive, dead, wholly imagined—each having their input, each with their own radically different forms of being, each with their own suffering, each with a different stake in the outcome.

And they can all have a part to play.

The "patient" is, evidently, the person sitting in front of us—that person, right there—the one who wants to be fixed.

The "patient" is a whole world of interdependent, suffering people—and we are part of that cast.

I guess my minimal claim is this: That to be explicitly open to this, and aware, will make us better, as doctors, in almost every way. And life will be infinitely more interesting.

I wish you all the best,
Peter

CHAPTER

7

Steps toward
Deep Listening

Ronald M. Epstein

> *"You're listening to what I'm saying to you, not just hearing, there's a big difference between listening and hearing somebody. You can hear a noise and not pay attention to it. But if you listen to it, you can figure out what it is. So, that's what I want them to do, listen to what I'm saying."*
>
> **Patient from focus group about respect in healthcare (Beach et al., 2017)**

> *"The capacity to give one's attention to a sufferer is a very rare and difficult thing; it is almost a miracle; it is a miracle. Nearly all those who think they have this capacity do not possess it."*
>
> **Simone Weil (Weil & Soskice, 2021)**

Prologue

I saw "Kevin"[1] on my schedule in my family medicine clinic. Over the past decade I had helped him navigate the complexities of heart disease, depression, and a shaky marriage; we knew each other well and had a good relationship. After sitting down and a warm greeting, Kevin was direct: "I've always really liked you as a doctor, but ever since you got this new computer system, I feel that you just haven't been listening as well. Thought I should tell you."

DOI: 10.1201/9781003593294-7

I felt devastated. I knew it was true; the electronic health record (EHR) had hijacked my attention. Its clumsy platform, byzantine algorithms, and incessant alerts had depleted my ability to stay focused on what really mattered to my patients—and to me. Unknowingly, my survival strategy was to privilege instrumental tasks over relational ones. Even worse, I had taught communication skills for my whole career, to medical students, residents, and practicing doctors, and now this; I had failed at the very thing that I was teaching.

I allowed myself a momentary pause to gather my thoughts. As my defensiveness dissipated, I realized that this was not only "distracted doctoring" (Papadakos & Bertman, 2017); it was also about my identity as a healer and about working in a broken healthcare system. The only thing that made sense was to say, "Thank you," expressing gratitude for his courage to point out the costs of technology and for providing motivation to change my relationship with it.

The kind of listening Kevin wanted—and that I wanted—was more than hearing Kevin's words. Listening involved attentively privileging the most important things—understanding and honouring Kevin's lived experience, building a relationship, and organizing the medical tasks to be navigated during the visit—all in the context of addressing the implicit and explicit demands of a healthcare enterprise oriented towards productivity and transaction rather than healing and relationship. Listening involved choices when and how to listen and judgements about what was most important. It was stunning for me to realize that, in the moments I was looking at the screen rather than listening to Kevin, I wasn't attending to that which was most important to Kevin, and to me. I had been unaware.

I knew I had to do something. The first word that came to mind was "mini-rebellion." Rather than habitually opening the EHR as soon as I arrived in the patient's room (as I had been instructed to do), I decided to try an experiment. For the first minute or 90 seconds of each patient visit I would just listen, starting with an invitation for the patient to begin. If I didn't understand something, I'd ask for clarification, and when called for, I'd indicate understanding and support. Importantly, I'd just listen and wait 90 seconds before interrupting, interpreting, diagnosing, or giving advice.

It didn't take long for my mini-rebellion to lead to feeling a certain lightness of being that had been missing since the new EHR came on the scene. I noticed that I didn't need to repeat questions because I actually listened to the answer the first time. I was present, not just going through the motions, not just phoning it in. My chart notes were more focused and actionable. And I didn't get home any later than usual after a busy day. My mini-rebellion was a moral act. It redefined my relationship to technology. Although the healthcare system valued productivity and documentation rather than human understanding, I didn't have to abide by those values. The realization that my actions reflected that I, too, was complicit with values that deviated from my own was unsettling. I needed to take action, for myself and my patients, and for the medical enterprise as a whole.

My background and motivations for being a doctor are relevant here. As a child I was asthmatic, visiting doctors frequently in an era when treatments were largely ineffective, understanding what it was like to be ill and, fortunately, what it was like to be treated with kindness and respect by caring doctors. My path to medical school was indirect: I graduated from university with a music degree, and during various digressions in my studies, hitchhiked from Greece to Norway, drove a taxicab in Manhattan on the night shift to pay for my studies, studied traditional Chinese medicine, and took up a Zen meditation practice. Only in retrospect did it become clear to me these were all connected. Music, meditation, conversing with "rides," and meeting people during my travels who, with kindness, took me into their homes, were all opportunities to listen to myself and to others and to have raw unfiltered experience of the world. After university, while studying abroad, two illness experiences that put me in touch with the lived experience of suffering set me on a path back to my childhood aspiration to be a doctor.

Although I had many inspired teachers, I found medical school to be intellectually lacking and lacking attention to what was human and humane in caring for those who suffer. The mentors who had the greatest positive impact on me were at the margins of the institutional enterprise. One wisely directed me to bio-psychosocially oriented postgraduate training opportunities at the University of Rochester in 1984, where I have remained since, with 35 years working in community-based primary care overlapping with 17 years in hospital-based palliative care. Knowing from the beginning that the most rewarding aspects of doctoring involved the relational aspects of care, these became my teaching and research focus. I worked with patients with AIDS in the early years of the epidemic before effective treatments were available, then with other groups of patients with serious and incurable illnesses. I developed and taught courses in communication skills for learners at all levels and workshops on mindful practice and self-awareness for experienced doctors, nurses, and researchers. Both in education and research, I have had to confront the vestiges of an outdated worldview that rigidly separates the biological and the relational (Engel, 1992).

What Patients Want and Need

Movies, TV, podcasts, storytellers, fictional accounts, and the medical literature regularly feature accounts in which the doctor doesn't listen well, sometimes with devastating consequences. While many of these issues are not new (modern "scientific" medicine has been critiqued for privileging an objectivist/biological stance for at least 100 years, and even Plato provides examples of physicians who listen well and individualize care and those who don't), the context has changed. For example, corporatization of medicine in the United States and some other countries increasingly prioritizes clinical productivity, through-put, and superficial quality metrics that largely exclude human relationships from the conceptual map.

Preparing to write this chapter, I combed the medical literature about listening in healthcare contexts. Although research on effective communication has blossomed in the past 30 years, I could find very few research studies focusing on listening. What I did find were dozens of personal narratives about when listening didn't happen or went awry. These accounts converge on patients' basic needs and expectations from doctors: To be respected, heard, and known as a person; to be and feel understood; to have their concerns considered valid and important; to trust that the doctor prioritizes the patient's needs over their own and has the expertise to care for them; and to support and to advocate for patients to live a full and meaningful life, achieving health-related outcomes that they value (McWhinney, 1997). Listening stood at the centre of establishing a therapeutic relationship, managing strong emotions and uncertainty, sharing information, achieving shared understanding, making decisions, and helping patients take an active role in their healthcare (Epstein & Street, 2007). Patients and their families know that listening builds connection and trust between doctor and patient through a sense of presence, feeling seen and known, in contrast to an ethos of detached concern (Candib, 2002; Charon, 2017; Jagosh et al., 2011; Kishton et al., 2023)—even if cure or reversal of disease is not possible. Small efforts matter; in one study, patients were more satisfied if the doctor listened to at least three uninterrupted sentences early in the consultation (Tallman et al., 2007), hardly an insurmountable task, yet a rarity (Marvel et al., 1999).

Listening has moral value, and its absence is a moral failure. Physician-philosopher Eric Cassell described how *the only way to learn . . . whether suffering is present is to ask the sufferer*" and to listen to the response (Cassell, 1982). The moral failure of not listening becomes more real to health professionals when they are on the receiving end of healthcare. Near the end of her life, my mother, 88 years old, with moderate dementia, in hospice care for advanced stage IV lung cancer and dependent on oxygen, sustained a hip fracture. Despite my having informed the hospital team that she was terminally ill and unfit to tolerate major surgery, the orthopaedic team prepared for a total hip replacement, because it would be "the treatment of choice for femoral neck fractures," ignoring the contextual factors that I had communicated. Only after demanding a meeting with the internal medicine, palliative care, and orthopaedic surgery teams present was the procedure was aborted, and she was provided adequate pain relief to spend her final days at home.

Listening is both an expectation and a gift. Like many doctors, periodically I receive letters of gratitude from patients. Few mention accurate diagnoses and wise selection of medications; nearly all talk about presence, attentiveness, listening, and caring. Listening confers respect, especially important for those who are minoritized, stigmatized, and discounted and who have difficulty navigating the healthcare system due to low literacy, poor access, and disparate cultural norms. Listening also promotes health professionals' satisfaction and well-being.

Facets of Listening

Early in training, doctors learn that clinical conversations are different from social conversations (Epstein & Beach, 2023). Effective listening in medical settings involves attention to biomedical tasks, human relationships, and context. When task-focused, patient and doctor clarify clinical details to arrive at a diagnosis and move toward a treatment plan. When focusing on relationships, the goals are achieving shared understanding; honouring patients' values, concerns, beliefs, and emotions; and communicating trust and respect, considering that patients often are fearful and apprehensive and power dynamics are paramount. Contextual listening takes a wide-angle view of the patient's life, recognizing that the meanings of, and responses to, illness are conditioned by the patient's family, social supports, finances, education, and literacy and that contacts between doctors and patients are episodic, brief, and information-rich (Weiner, 2022). These three facets are all necessary to create a sense of shared mind in which clinicians' efforts align with what matters most to patients (Epstein, 2013). Yet, in training, doctors learn to privilege task-focused listening as the "main course," relegating relational and contextual listening to "side dishes."

Silence can also create connection (Bartels et al., 2016). A brief pause or an extended silence can communicate powerful emotions and reactions. Silences are not all the same; as a clinician, I listen for—and respond to—expectant silences, awkward silences, compassionate silences, and eloquent silences. And I create silences through pauses when I speak to make room for patients' voices, to acknowledge a message that can be communicated best by silence, and to share the spaciousness of silence itself.

Listening to Myself

As a musician, I listen to myself in three ways. I listen to my intention—I hear the notes before I play them, an imaginative construction of the music I intend to create. Then, I listen to the sounds as they come out of the instrument with an aesthetic ear, enjoying the sensual experience, and a critical ear, making micro-adjustments and improvisations to lend coherence to a phrase. Finally, I listen as if I were in the audience, imagining the sound and emotional experience of the audience.

When I'm with patients I listen to myself in similar ways. On a concrete level, I listen to my intentions—what I hope might happen during the visit, my words, and the received effect of my communication. But listening to myself is deeper than that; it is an opportunity to be aware of my predispositions, biases, and expectations and my own state of mind: *Am I being attentive? Open? Curious? In the face of uncertainty or conflict, am I feeling defensive? Am I able to set aside judgement and categorization until the patient has had their say? Am I able to adopt a frame of reference in which patients' concerns make sense and are actionable? Am I willing to learn?*

Before meeting a patient, I prepare mentally to focus my attention. Seeing a patient's name, age, and presenting symptoms on an office schedule invites speculation about who the patient is, what the diagnosis might be, and what treatment the doctor might offer. Consider William, an older male with a "urinary problem." Even before seeing him, I find myself beginning to construct one or more plausible stories, including a diagnosis (e.g., worsening prostate problem), treatment (e.g., medication), and referral (e.g., to urology). Sometimes these hunches are accurate or at least create a frame, a starting point. However, when hunches lead to prematurely categorizing a patient, I am at risk. I might stop listening, ask questions just to confirm my presuppositions, or unknowingly exclude from consideration biomedical (e.g., medication side effect) and contextual factors (e.g., proximity of the bathroom in the workplace). When I am practising at my best, I maintain a "beginner's mind" so that I can be open to alternative ways of under-standing a clinical situation, even changing my mind, and, in the face of uncertainty, holding more than one perspective at a time.

Recognizing that reflective self-awareness is rarely part of clinical training, I felt it important to put it on the map, and in 1999, my article, "Mindful Practice," defined qualities of expert clinicians—including attentive obser-vation, curiosity, beginner's mind, and presence—that help them adopt moment-to-moment self-awareness during everyday work with the goal of greater clarity, compassion, competence, and clinical wisdom (Epstein, 1999). By making self-awareness an explicit task of medicine and medi-cal education, clinicians could more readily identify and build upon their strengths and positive attributes and be aware of and retool habits that impair listening, such as judgemental attitudes and premature closure, and avoid concerns that make the clinician feel uncomfortable. A body of research now confirms that mindfulness matters. Patients of doctors who are more mindful report greater trust, better communication, and more satisfactory relationships (Beach et al., 2013), and workshops focus-ing on mindful practice and deep listening improve physician well-being, satisfaction, and provision of compassionate patient-centred care (Epstein et al., 2022).

Not Listening

Steven Covey, author of the bestseller, *Seven Habits of Highly Effective People*, offered words of caution that *"Most people don't listen to understand, they lis-ten to respond"* (Covey, 1993). Doctors learn to think quickly. Listening to respond is implicitly reinforced. Doctors typically take control of clinical conversations within seconds (Rhoades et al., 2001), shaping the questions asked, missing opportunities to acknowledge patients' fears and emotions (Morse et al., 2008), and avoiding stigmatized topics (Epstein et al., 1998) When providing information, doctors rarely check that the information has been understood and assimilated, or even that it was desired in the first place. Doctors often adopt a "lecturing style" (rather than a more interac-tive back-and-forth style) which, although filled with information, hinders shared understanding (Ali et al., 2021).

Listening is not merely an individual matter; listening is relational and embedded in a medical enterprise with implicit values and norms. Stressed and sleep-deprived patients and clinical staff often interact in noisy, cha-otic, and understaffed environments, impairing everyone's "executive attention"—the ability to tune out distractions to focus on what's important (Epstein, 2017b). Unrealistic workloads and meaningless administrative tasks crowd out time that could be devoted to listening to and responding to patients' concerns. EHRs can compound the problem by directing doctors' attention to the screen rather than the patient, inviting them to privilege information in the chart rather a patient's first-person account (Verghese, 2008).

Patients and their care partners also have a role. Even when clinicians work hard to establish trust, patients might engage in "selective sharing" of information based on what they believe others would find relevant (Kehoe et al., 2022), avoid disclosing potentially stigmatizing information, respond with avoidance or anger when clinicians raise sensitive topics, and be reluctant to express their disagreements with the doctor's approach (Adams et al., 2012).

Learning to Listen

Deep listening can take many forms. In my primary care practice, I cared for "Joyce," a woman with distressing and sometimes incapacitating chronic abdominal pain for over 20 years. Her physical examination and diagnostic tests revealed no clues as to the cause. Numerous specialists were stumped. She entered psychotherapy, which was helpful, yet the pain persisted. One day, though, she seemed different in a way I found it difficult to characterize. It would have been so easy to consider this "more of the same." But I noticed that she used different gestures and words when describing her pain. In my uncertainty, I was both curious and worried. I did a careful physical examination and, feeling something suspicious, I suggested yet another scan, which revealed an ovarian cancer, the early diagnosis making treatment more feasible. Listening to her (her choice of words and gestures) and myself (my rising worry) made the difference. For me, the message was clear; adopting a "beginner's mind," not letting expertise and expectations get in the way of maintaining an openness to possibility, helped to avoid the deceptions arising from unexamined prior experience. Beginner's mind, in this case, was an attitude of "not knowing," tempering certainty with healthy self-doubt. Reflecting further, I had engaged in self-questioning, asking, "What am I assuming that might not be true?" and "What might I not be hearing?" (Epstein, 2017a).

At the height of the COVID-19 pandemic, Rana Awdish, a pulmonology colleague working in critical care, authored a moving article about a highly charged conflict with a patient whom she had known for more than a decade. Coming for a routine office visit, the patient ripped off her mask and invited her doctor to do the same, ranting about how COVID was a hoax and a "money-making scheme" (Adawi Awdish, 2021). Awdish was initially enraged. She describes, however, that in taking a momentary pause, she could gain "a millimeter's worth" of distance between her anger and her deeper values of understanding and compassion. She continues, "I allowed myself to move toward her, and her face reemerged. I sat down across from her and said only what was true, *'I do have a desire to protect myself based on what I've seen, and I will be keeping the mask on. And I wonder, what has this experience been like for you?'*" Expressing solidarity and vulnerability, she continues: "*'I wish I could make this all go away, for both of us,'* I offered, my voice shaking. *'More than anything I wish that.'* I pressed the backs of my hands up to my eyes to push back the visions and memorials and agonizing denial. *'The losses I've seen have been unbearable.'*"

Only then did the patient talk about her fears, and her loneliness, having been excluded from family events because she refused to observe precautions, and, only then, could they chart a path forward. Awdish's article brings into sharp relief the need for "epistemic reciprocity" (Dell'Olio et al., 2023; Kidd & Carel, 2017), a sincere belief that what another person says is valuable and giving them the attention they deserve. Its opposite is epistemic injustice. Not only differing belief systems, but "broken" English, strong body odours, lack of employment, fear, mistrust, and anger can lead clinicians to assume that a patient is "unintelligent," "demanding," "difficult," "crazy," or "non-compliant"—until the clinician listens. Awdish's approach reflects what psychologist Rollo May describes as "a capacity to pause and, in that pause, to choose the one response toward which we wish to throw our weight" (May, 1975). He continues, "The capacity to create ourselves, based upon this freedom, is inseparable from consciousness or self-awareness."

Early in my medical career, just as I was finishing training, I cared for "Bob," a middle-aged man hospitalized with near-fatal complications of alcoholic hepatitis who experienced an unexpected and complete recovery. I grew to know him over the ensuing 25 years. Extroverted, garrulous, and grateful to be alive, he came to be a favourite of the staff at the clinic. Typically, he would chat with people in the office about details of their personal lives, where they lived, their families, and what they enjoyed. Living alone and estranged from his ex-wife and two daughters, he wanted to reconnect with them and get his life together. Shortly after he started psychotherapy, his therapist called, telling me that Bob had shared important information with her that

I should know. Going through the possibilities in my mind, I never considered what was to come; much earlier in his life, Bob had been a hit man for the Mafia, having learned "the business" from his father. He had killed eight and maimed several others, never having been caught. He wanted me to know, too. In my initial panic, I ascertained that there was no one at current risk (including me) and that I had no legal obligations to report. I struggled to listen and be present in a way that had previously been effortless; suddenly, I was seeing him through a different lens—of ambivalence, assumptions, and fear. He knew where I lived. The only path that made sense, though, was one of moving towards dissonance, holding the seemingly contradictory images of him as a sweet and caring man who could bring joy to others, a grateful patient, a suffering person struggling with demons, a recovering addict, and a criminal. It took some effort for me to again see his humanity and to see him as courageous in his seeking that which most humans want—love, connection, healing, and understanding. Living with those contradictory images without trying to reconcile them was instrumental in reducing my fear and defensiveness and helped me to listen.

Learning to listen might paradoxically be enhanced by the same technologies that inhibit it. About 10 years ago, I was approached by Ehsan Hoque, a computer science colleague at my university. He was interested in how computers could help people communicate with one another more effectively. As a digital immigrant, I was baffled how this could be true. He continued. As the guardian of his brother who has autism, Ehsan developed a program for autistic young adults to help them communicate with others in a more effective way. He developed technology whereby a human could have a spoken conversation with an on-screen avatar and receive computer-generated feedback on communication style. He wanted to apply the same technology to conversations doctors have with seriously ill patients, those nearing the end of life. I was dubious, until he demonstrated that the same program could analyse audio-recorded conversations between seriously ill patients and their doctors and discover patterns of communication that human coders had missed entirely. Two patterns emerged that were closely associated with patient understanding of the severity of their illness—using a back-and-forth interactional style rather than a more typical unidirectional lecturing style and emotional variability in speech rather than a dry "professional" tone (Ali et al., 2021). These findings resonated strongly with me; he had discovered manifestations of power dynamics and the "clinical gaze." He then created an on-screen affect-sensitive conversational partner, an avatar portraying a woman with advanced cancer; driven by large language models, the computer could rapidly assess communication dynamics and provide specific feedback to the doctor interacting with the program about turn-taking, emotional trajectory, empathic communication, use of clear language, and helping the patient give voice to what was important to them. Recently, the program demonstrated improvements in the quality of the doctor's subsequent communication (Haut et al., 2023). For me, it was mind-bending to imagine that a computer program could achieve this level of specificity and influence on behaviours that we identify as essentially human and could offer a means for helping doctors be self-aware and communicate more effectively—and humanely.

There are words behind the words. Learning to listen involves not just listening to *what* patients say, but *when* and *why* they say it (Schegloff & Sacks, 1973). Some of this happens intuitively. *The other doctor gave me a cream but didn't tell me how long I am supposed to use it?* is a question to be answered rather than a statement of fact. But sometimes it requires active attention and questioning. Let's say a patient asks, *Will I have to take this medication for the rest of my life?* Is this a request for information? Or is it a way of saying that they are struggling to accept a new reality that threatens their identity as a healthy person (McArthur, 2023)? A reminder to avoid over-concreteness.

Doctors who are attentive and present with patients tend to respond with authenticity and sincerity, not merely "phoning it in." A few years ago, I was seen in the emergency room with severe abdominal pain. The care I received was technically excellent, but the moment I remember the most vividly was when the person transporting me on a gurney to the CT scanner stopped momentarily, looked me in the eye, and asked, "How are you doing?" And he listened for the answer. With four of his words, I felt cared for. But what happens when doctors don't *feel* a connection with a patient or find it difficult to listen? "Presentational" skills, engaging in "deep acting" with the intention of building trust and connection (Larson & Yao, 2005), might be second-best. But there are dangers; distressed patients may see through the act and leave feeling unsatisfied with their care (Yagil & Shnapper-Cohen, 2016).

Finally, patients want to know that they are being listened to. Here, sitting down, eye contact, leaning forward, tone of voice, and other forms of non-verbal and paraverbal communication are paramount (Little et al., 2015; Robertson, 2005). Responding to emotional cues (e.g., "Are you worried?"), clarifying understanding ("Do I have this right?"), invitations ("Tell me more."), and curiosity ("What happened next?") signpost that one is listening and do not increase consultation time (Coulehan et al., 2001; Platt et al., 2001).

A Path Forward

These anecdotes only represent a few points in the complexity of human communication. Yet they tickle the imagination about what is possible. There are some caveats. Asking trainees and seasoned clinicians to bring openness and curiosity to their interactions with patients can also raise a sense of vulnerability, inadequacy, shame, or deviance. As a medical student on the internal medicine service, I was caring for what the house staff called a "fascinoma," a patient whose disease was one of the first for which the pathophysiology could be understood on a genetic/molecular level. Caring for her, I saw a lonely old woman whose pain was being neglected and whom nobody visited. I recall the sense of fear and vulnerability in raising an observation to the house staff that might not be well received. Fortunately, this time it had a good outcome. I mentioned that pain medications might help, which the house staff provided. Yet it took a medical student to bring them to listen to what she had been saying, not merely hearing it. Often such situations don't end up well and invite defensiveness and shaming rather than gratitude and camaraderie.

As educators we can do better. Introducing students to the palliative care service, I emphasize that there are four "patients" when I'm doing a consultation: The person in the bed, their family and support network, the (often distressed) clinicians who are asking for the consultation, and me. All four "patients" need listening, attention, and healing, and we discuss each as part of each case discussion. To create a sense of shared vulnerability, I share what I know and what I don't, where I get stuck, and how I muddle through seemingly impossible situations—and encourage the learner to do the same.

The culture of medicine is a collection of conversations and practices—what the protagonists notice, hear, and listen for. The way clinicians listen is a manifestation of macro-structures that place value on some conversations and not on others. Yet clinicians who have had the experience of being listened to might be more likely to listen deeply to their patients. Discussion groups about difficult moments in clinical care, individual coaching sessions focusing on communication, relationships and teamwork, and peer support programs for when unexpected or untoward events occur are increasingly available. These provide an avenue for greater psychological safety to listen and be present amid complexity, chaos, uncertainty, and strong emotions. At a large New York City hospital, the head of the neurosurgery department has instituted a "mindful pause" before starting every surgical procedure. First, they establish the basics—the right patient, the right procedure, the right side—then, in the mindful pause, a reminder about who the patient is as a person—their family, the impact of the illness—and an invitation for all who are participating in the procedure to listen and be present with one another and with the patient during and after the procedure. This was initially seen as a radical move and now is embedded in the culture of the department.

It would be naïve to suggest that changing long-standing communicational habits that are continually reinforced in medical culture is a small task. Yet it is possible to develop listening skills (Boudreau et al., 2009) and employ them in highly stressful and chaotic clinical environments. And, at the organizational level, good listening should be monitored as a marker of high-quality care, enacted by leaders, and a focus of clinical education and research.

Acknowledgments

I thank Mary Catherine Beach for her contributions to the published article upon which some of the content of this chapter is based. Richard Street, Jr. provided insights into the nuances of presentational skills, deep acting, empathy, and deep listening. Amanda McArthur provided yet-unpublished findings on the application of conversation analysis to the art of listening. Iona Health and Caroline Engen provided insightful critique of early drafts of this chapter.

Note

1 All names have been changed to respect confidentiality.

References

Adams, J. R., Elwyn, G., Legare, F., & Frosch, D. L. (2012). Communicating with physicians about medical decisions: A reluctance to disagree. *Archives of Internal Medicine*, 1–2. https://doi.org/10.1001/archinternmed.2012.2360[pii][doi]. (Not in File)
Adawi Awdish, R. L. (2021). You don't ever let go of the thread. *Annals of Internal Medicine*, 174(11), 1628–1629.
Ali, M. R., Sen, T., Kane, B., Bose, S., Carroll, T., Epstein, R. M., Schubert, L. K., & Hoque, E. (2021). Novel computational linguistic measures, dialogue system and the development of SOPHIE: Standardized online patient for healthcare interaction education. *IEEE Transactions on Affective Computing*. https://doi.org/10.1109/TAFFC.2021.3054717

Bartels, J., Rodenbach, R., Ciesinski, K., Gramling, R., Fiscella, K., & Epstein, R. (2016). Eloquent silences: A musical and lexical analysis of conversation between oncologists and their patients. *Patient Education and Counseling, 99*(10), 1584–1594. https://doi.org/10.1016/j.pec.2016.04.009

Beach, M. C., Branyon, E., & Saha, S. (2017). Diverse patient perspectives on respect in healthcare: A qualitative study. *Patient Education and Counseling, 100*(11), 2076–2080. https://doi.org/10.1016/j.pec.2017.05.010

Beach, M. C., Roter, D., Korthuis, P. T., Epstein, R. M., Sharp, V., Ratanawongsa, N., Cohn, J., Eggly, S., Sankar, A., Moore, R. D., & Saha, S. (2013). A multicenter study of physician mindfulness and health care quality. *The Annals of Family Medicine, 11*(5), 421–428. https://doi.org/10.1370/afm.1507

Boudreau, J. D., Cassell, E., & Fuks, A. (2009). Preparing medical students to become attentive listeners. *Medical Teacher, 31*(1), 22–29. https://doi.org/10.1080/01421590802350776

Candib, L. M. (2002). Working with suffering. *Patient Education and Counseling, 48*(1), 43–50. http://dx.doi.org/10.1016/S0738-3991%2802%2900098-8

Cassell, E. J. (1982). The nature of suffering and the goals of medicine. *New England Journal of Medicine, 306*(11), 639–645. (In File)

Charon, R. (2017). To see the suffering. *Academic Medicine, 92*(12), 1668–1670. https://doi.org/10.1097/acm.0000000000001989

Coulehan, J. L., Platt, F. W., Egener, B., Frankel, R., Lin, C. T., Lown, B., & Salazar, W. H. (2001). "Let me see if I have this right . . .": Words that help build empathy. *Annals of Internal Medicine, 135*(3), 221–227. http://www.ncbi.nlm.nih.gov/pubmed/11487497 (Not in File)

Covey, S. R. (1993). *The seven habits of highly effective people.* Fireside.

Dell'Olio, M., Whybrow, P., & Reeve, J. (2023). Examining the knowledge work of person-centred care: Towards epistemic reciprocity. *Patient Education and Counseling, 107,* 107575. https://doi.org/10.1016/j.pec.2022.107575

Engel, G. L. (1992). How much longer must medicine's science be bound by a seventeenth century world view? *Psychotherapy and Psychosomatics, 57*(1–2), 3–16.

Epstein, R. M. (1999). Mindful practice. *JAMA, 282*(9), 833–839. https://doi.org/10.1001/jama.282.9.833

Epstein, R. M. (2013). Whole mind and shared mind in clinical decision-making. *Patient Education and Counseling, 90*(2), 200–206. https://doi.org/10.1016/j.pec.2012.06.035

Epstein, R. M. (2017a). *Attending: Medicine, mindfulness, and humanity.* Scribner.

Epstein, R. M. (2017b). Mindful practitioners, mindful teams, and mindful organizations: Attending to the core tasks of medicine. In P. J. Papadakos & S. Bertman (Eds.), *Distracted doctoring: Returning to patient-centered care in the digital age* (pp. 229–243). Springer International Publishing AG. https://doi.org/10.1007/978-3-319-48707-6

Epstein, R. M., & Beach, M. C. (2023). "I don't need your pills, I need your attention": Steps toward deep listening in medical encounters. *Current Opinion in Psychology,* 101685.

Epstein, R. M., Marshall, F., Sanders, M., & Krasner, M. S. (2022). Effect of an intensive mindful practice workshop on patient-centered compassionate care, clinician well-being, work engagement, and teamwork. *Journal of Continuing Education in the Health Professions, 42*(1), 19–27. https://doi.org/10.1097/ceh.0000000000000379

Epstein, R. M., Morse, D. S., Frankel, R. M., Frarey, L., Anderson, K., & Beckman, H. B. (1998). Awkward moments in patient-physician communication about HIV risk. *Annals of Internal Medicine, 128*(6), 435–442. (In File)

Epstein, R. M., & Street, R. L., Jr. (2007). *Patient-centered communication in cancer care: Promoting healing and reducing suffering.* National Cancer Institute, NIH. http://www. outcomes.cancer.gov/areas/pcc/communication/monograph.html

Haut, K., Wohn, C., Kane, B., Carroll, T., Guigno, C., Kumar, V., Epstein, R., Schubert, L., & Hoque, E. (2023). Validating a virtual human and automated feedback system for training doctor-patient communication skills. *Proceedings of Affective Computing and Intelligent Interaction (ACII) Conference.* https://doi.org/10.48550/arXiv.2306.15213(arXiv)

Jagosh, J., Donald Boudreau, J., Steinert, Y., MacDonald, M. E., & Ingram, L. (2011). The importance of physician listening from the patients' perspective: Enhancing diagnosis, healing, and the doctor–patient relationship. *Patient Education and Counseling, 85*(3), 369–374. https://doi.org/10.1016/j.pec.2011.01.028

Kehoe, L., Sanapala, C., DiGiovanni, G., Yousefi-Nooraie, R., Yilmaz, S., Bauer, J., Loh, K. P., Norton, S., Duberstein, P., Kamen, C., Gilmore, N., Gudina, A., Kleckner, A., Mohile, S., & Epstein, R. M. (2022). Older adults with advanced cancer are selective in sharing and seeking information with social networks. *Patient Education and Counseling, 105*(10), 3116–3122. https://doi.org/10.1016/j.pec.2022.06.005

Kidd, I. J., & Carel, H. (2017). Epistemic Injustice and Illness. *Journal of Applied Philosophy, 34*(2), 172–190. https://doi.org/10.1111/japp.12172

Kishton, R., Patel, H., Saini, D., Millstein, J., & Levy, A. (2023). Listening as medicine: A thematic analysis. *Patient Experience Journal, 10*(1), 64–71.

Larson, E. B., & Yao, X. (2005). Clinical empathy as emotional labor in the patient-physician relationship. *JAMA, 293*(9), 1100–1106. http://www.ncbi.nlm.nih.gov/pubmed/15741532 (Not in File)

Little, P., White, P., Kelly, J., Everitt, H., & Mercer, S. (2015). Randomised controlled trial of a brief intervention targeting predominantly non-verbal communication in general practice consultations. *The British Journal of General Practice, 65*(635), e351–e356. https://doi.org/10.3399/bjgp15X685237

Marvel, M. K., Epstein, R. M., Flowers, K., & Beckman, H. B. (1999). Soliciting the patient's agenda: Have we improved? *JAMA, 281*(3), 283–287. http://www.ncbi.nlm.nih.gov/pubmed/9918487 (Not in File)

May, R. (1975). *The courage to create.* Bantam.

McArthur, A. W. (2023). *When patients push back: Patient resistance to diagnostic closure in primary care.* Society of General Internal Medicine.

McWhinney, I. R. (1997). Illness, suffering, and healing. In I. R. McWhinney (Ed.), *A textbook of family medicine* (2nd ed., pp. 83–103). Oxford University Press.

Morse, D. S., Edwardsen, E. A., & Gordon, H. S. (2008). Missed opportunities for interval empathy in lung cancer communication. *Archives of Internal Medicine, 168*(17), 1853–1858. http://www.ncbi.nlm.nih.gov/pubmed/18809811 (Not in File)

Papadakos, P. J., & Bertman, S. (2017). *Distracted doctoring: Returning to patient-centered care in the digital age.* Springer.

Platt, F. W., Gaspar, D. L., Coulehan, J. L., Fox, L., Adler, A. J., Weston, W. W., Smith, R. C., & Stewart, M. (2001). "Tell me about yourself": The patient-centered interview. *Annals of Internal Medicine, 134*(11), 1079–1085. (In File)

Rhoades, D. R., McFarland, K. F., Finch, W. H., & Johnson, A. O. (2001). Speaking and interruptions during primary care office visits. *Family Medicine, 33*(7), 528–532. http://www.ncbi.nlm.nih.gov/pubmed/11456245 (Not in File)

Robertson, K. (2005). Active listening: More than just paying attention [other journal article]. *Australian Family Physician, 34*(12). https://search.informit.org/doi/10.3316/informit.366629010280498

Schegloff, E., & Sacks, H. (1973). Opening up closings. *Semiotica, 8*(4), 289–327. https://doi.org/10.1515/semi.1973.8.4.289

Tallman, K., Janisse, T., Frankel, R. M., Sung, S. H., Krupat, E., & Hsu, J. T. (2007). Communication practices of physicians with high patient-satisfaction ratings. *The Permanente Journal, 11*(1), 19.

Verghese, A. (2008). Culture shock—patient as icon, icon as patient. *The New England Journal of Medicine, 359*(26), 2748–2751.

Weil, S., & Soskice, J. (2021). *Waiting for God (1950)*. Routledge.

Weiner, S. J. (2022). Contextualizing care: An essential and measurable clinical competency. *Patient Education and Counseling, 105*(3), 594–598.

Yagil, D., & Shnapper-Cohen, M. (2016). When authenticity matters most: Physicians' regulation of emotional display and patient satisfaction. *Patient Education and Counseling, 99*(10), 1694–1698. https://doi.org/10.1016/j.pec.2016.04.003

Your Everyday—My Once in a Lifetime

Knut Eirik Eliassen

Texting: *Hey! How are you? When was it I was supposed to pick you up for training? Love, Dad*

- No answer

Are you ok?

- No answer

You good? I'll pick you up at half past 4. Dad

- No answer

- Starting to worry a little, but shake it off.

- Time passes—closing in to pick-up time.

"PLING"—"I'm in the ER"

You're what! Are you kidding?

- Tries to call—No answer

Yeah, I fell on my bike. Are you home?

Not anymore—I'm on my way up to you. I'll be there in 10.

The pictures in my head comprise a bloody face, knocked-out teeth, and, gratefully, a bicycle helmet—at least I think so.

- Enter the hospital, where I used to work. Go to the waiting room for the out-of-hour services, where I've picked up patients myself on more than 100 calls. There's no Bjørn here.

DOI: 10.1201/9781003593294-8

- Go to the reception—they know who I am. *"Hey, I got a call from my son."*

- *"Yes, he's in here, follow me."*

I find a pale young man lying on a stretcher with his jacket still on and a woollen blanket around his legs. He smiles briefly, looks at his teacher. *"Hi—I'm Bjørn's dad. Thanks for driving him and staying here. What happened?"*

"He can tell you himself, but we couldn't make him stand up, so I got my car, and these other students helped me to get him up. Arriving here, we couldn't make him stand either, so the nurses got him a wheelchair. Good luck, now, I understand he's in good hands with you, so if it's OK, I'll leave."

"Yes, sure, thanks again. We'll keep you posted."

The teacher leaves, and I go over to my 16 year old and give him a big hug—the biggest I dare, given the potential extent of his injuries. He moans, cries, fixes on a brave face, and gets his colour back.

"OK, you. Tell me what happened." And he tells me that he was on his way home together with a pal. He biked a little bit faster than what was smart in the school yard and looked back at the friend while talking. All of a sudden, a sidewalk came close and instead of jumping onto it, he instinctively hit the brakes, then just fell onto the curb with the bike over him. A sudden pain, and after that he wasn't able to get up again. *"Does it still hurt?"*

"Yes."

"They give you something?"

"I got a paracetamol, I think, just before you arrived."

"OK—let me take a look at you."

I do a quick trauma examination. His head, spine, and belly are fine, as is the right leg. Bruised on the left hip and calf. No larger bleedings. Normal distal sensibility of the left leg, moves his toes, but is not able to move the hip or knee because of pain.

So far, so good. And yes—he had been wearing his helmet.

We need an x-ray of the hip. I look at my watch. If things are as they used to be around here, we are now in the middle of the change of who's on call. The day doctor leaves in 5 and the night shift is not on before 90 minutes unless something serious happens, and this is not serious enough. I am about to pull the string to get the nurse's attention when she comes through the door: *"Hi—how are you? Did the medication help you anything?"*

"Not sure."

"OK, I'll be off now, but the other nurse knows you're here, alright?"

"OK."

I dare to jump in with a question—*"Am I right, that we're in the middle of shifts now? I think he needs an x-ray. Could that be arranged for before the doctor leaves, you think?"*

"I'll see what I can do."

In a situation like this—time passes both fast and slowly. Now, half an hour goes by in a blink, and I know there is no doctor around to order the x-ray.

A new nurse arrives, checks briefly on Bjørn, and says—*"I'll see if I can get hold of a doctor for you."*

Shortly after, a young doctor arrives. Doesn't introduce herself, just says—*"So the hip, hah? I'll arrange for an x-ray."* No story, just lifts the blanket, concludes that it is the left side that is bruised. Touches the hip superficially and unstructured—just enough that it hurts. Says *"OK"* and turns around to wash her hands.

It is strange—she arranged for a request for an x-ray, which is what we asked for. Nevertheless, I am overwhelmed by an unwelcome emotion. A mix of hostility and *anger*—she sees my son, sees us, not necessarily as a burden, but at least as something not worth investing any time, empathy, or effort into. To us, this is a rare occasion, filled with worry and other negative emotions—a once-in-a-lifetime moment for us, really. Not much more than an hour ago, we were dealing with a completely normal everyday. All of a sudden we're here, yet you see us as a boring chore.

Although I know the answer to the question, I ask her: *"So— That means we can go to the x-ray department?"*

"Sure."

"And, when we get back, do we see you again, or are we then to go to the orthopaedic outpatient clinic?"

"No, no—you're going to the other guys—Now, you're out of my hands!" She lifts her hands up and leaves without saying goodbye. It is as if we hear a sigh of relief from her as she leaves the room.

"Thank you . . . I guess," I hear myself whispering.

I look to my son, who shrugs, grimaces—*"Whatever."*

As he can't stand up or walk, I just take the stretcher and start walking towards the x-ray department. I can't even remember if I told the nurse we were leaving. At the ward, the doors and the expedition are closed, but there is a phone number to call for those with errands out of hours. I am just about to call when I hear intense crying from inside the ward. Knowing that there's only one radiographer on call in the evenings, I await. Then we wait some more.

We wait another 20 minutes before a tearful five year old comes out with his broken arm and sweaty parents. Shortly after, the just-as-sweaty radiographer sticks her head out and says with an unfriendly expression on her face—*"And you are?"*

I tell her our errand.

"No"—she says—*"You're not on my list,"* then leaves.

Now Bjørn has to pee—which is not very easy when you're 16 years old, can't stand on your feet, and you are in the middle of a hospital corridor. I weigh my alternatives: If the hip's broken, it's broken. If it's not, I can't break it. And I can't see you peeing in a bottle in the middle of the waiting room. So, I carry my 120-pound teenager to the toilet. Luckily, I'm taller than him still, so lifting him by the armpits, we somehow manage. It hurts and takes a bit of swearing. And even those of you not having a prostate can probably imagine that relieving yourself while hanging in your dad's arms and having the door open is not easy. Nevertheless, Bjørn closes his eyes, relaxes the best he can, and manages. Little did we know that getting back on the stretcher would be even more painful. He doesn't think of it himself, but I am just happy to see that he didn't pee any blood.

By this time, his mother arrives to find us stumbling back from the toilet. Back at the waiting room, the radiographer sticks her head out again to tell us she still can't find us on her list. I ask her whether this shouldn't go electronically and if we are actually waiting for something—but by the end of my question her door is already shut again. I leave Bjørn with his mum and go back to the ER to check whether the x-ray has been requested at all. The secretary looks at her computer and concludes that yes, it was sent more than an hour ago. *"Well,"* I tell her. *"Since it hasn't been received, I think we need to resend the request."* She goes in, talks to the quick young doctor we had briefly seen earlier, and tells me that she had gone in and sent it again. Everything should be fine now.

Back at the waiting room, nothing more happens. That is, other patients are let in to take x-rays. After yet another half an hour, a familiar face appears in the hospital corridor. *"Hey,"* he says, *"You're here?"* It is Jonas, one of my specialty registrars in family medicine. I supervise him twice a month—and now he is on call at the out-of-hours service. He comes to check on Bjørn—*"Hi, chief! How are you?"* and greets Christina, *"Are you getting everything you need?"*

I tell him about our struggle of getting an x-ray.

"Hm. Come with me," he says.

I follow Jonas to the doctor's office. He can quickly see that the x-ray request had failed to be sent, twice. The young and quick doctor comes by, and Jonas asks her how she had ordered the x-ray. *"Well, you see,"* he says, *"You have to connect this computer to the hospital system logging in here, and then you have to transfer your document and resend it in here."*

"Oh"—she said—*"I didn't know that."*

"That's OK," Jonas says, *"You're new, right. So, I'll be your supervisor tonight—and these things may seem easy, but now, for*

instance, these guys have been waiting for the x-ray for more than two hours. It's important you know these things, and if you don't—ask."

"Well, nobody told me. I heard it didn't work, so I did it again."

"Yes, but you did the same thing again—and that didn't help either. And as far as I know you didn't check whether it had worked out."

"Look, I'll show you." And she sits down and manages to log in to order the x-ray. At one point the computer asks for a phone number, and she asks—*"Whose phone number do I put in here?"*

Then I say—to Jonas basically, because the young doctor never introduced herself to me—*"I always give the nurse's number here. Then I know they'll take the call, and they'll let me know if I need to know."*

The young doctor turns to me, looks at me for the first time, and says, v e r y s l o w l y, *"Eh—you work here too?"*

And Jonas replies *"Well, he used to. He's my supervisor, and I'm yours, so now the circle is closed."*

"PLING"—message successfully sent—it says, and I leave for Bjørn before I get to see the quick doctor blushing, hopefully realizing that arrogance and being cocksure isn't the best cover for insecurity and being a newcomer.

Back at the waiting room, the radiographer has already opened the door to let Bjørn in. *"Sorry about that,"* she says. *"I was just on my way over to the ER to check where your request had got stuck. And I didn't mean to be impolite before, it was just that these parents were yelling at me and then there were four patients at a time coming from the ward and I was just surprised to see you waiting for me without even being on my list."*

"That's OK," I say, *"I know you're the only radiographer on call. And it wasn't your fault."*

She automatically expects me to wait outside while taking the pictures, but I ask whether I might join her in the booth instead to be able to take a look at the images on the screen. She then realizes we have worked together before. We've looked for brain strokes and pulmonary embolisms together, sat together in front of these same screens. I can see that she wants to tell me more about how it feels to be under the pressure of being on call and that she thinks I will understand—but by the time the computer tells us the images are done processing, she also realizes that right now, I am not here for her, but only here as a dad—and I am really wondering whether this hip is broken or not.

> *"That doesn't look right,"* I mutter and point towards the curve of the hip on the left side.

> *"Well, I don't know"* she says—*"I'm just taking the pictures—we'll have to wait for the radiologist."*

She wishes us luck. Can't quite meet my eye. We leave for the ER and get a new room. And wait. A third nurse comes by and wants to know whether Bjørn wants more pain killers. He doesn't. As long as he lies still, he feels somewhat OK.

> We wait a bit longer, then a new face enters. She looks through the room, rests her gaze for a microsecond at each of us looking us in the eye. *"Hi—are you Bjørn?"*

> *"Mm."*

> *"I'm Anna—the resident doctor in orthopaedics. Hi—I'm Anna, you're mum? Hi, dad? I'm Anna. How are you all doing?"*

> *"Well, yeah, I mean—we're fine? I guess. But we want to find out whether the hip is broken or not."*

> *"Yes, I understand. We'll get to that, we also want to find out. So, Bjørn, I am sorry that I have to ask you again what you've already told other people, and I need to examine you again. Is that OK with you?"*

> *"I guess."*

> *"First of all—tell me what happened."*

> *"Well, I . . ."* And he proceeds to recount the story.

> *"Oh, that doesn't sound good. But wait a second when was this— three o'clock, and now it's eight. You must be exhausted!"*

> *"Well."*

> *"And hungry? And thirsty? Tell me, have you gotten anything to drink since you came here?"*

> *"Eeh. A little water for my tablets, that's all."*

> *"And mum and dad—you must be thirsty as well, right? You know what—wait a second."* She leaves. Comes back with lemonade

and three glasses, and five minutes later a nurse shows up with yogurt and a sandwich for Bjørn. *"It's OK to eat—we don't know exactly what's wrong with your hip yet, but we do know we won't put you to surgery tonight. Now, where were we?"* She takes his story. Then examines him thoroughly. Although in pain, Bjørn is completely relaxed. Answers with a clear voice and in whole sentences, even smiles and laughs a bit, and I would say speaks up more than he as a teenager normally does at home. And he is lying on the stretcher in only his boxers without being shy or pale and tells her exactly which movements hurt the most.

"OK," she says. *"Now I know a bit more. I have to confer with my seniors, but I also really would like you to be able to stand up. Is it OK if I give you a bit more of those painkillers and then come back in 20?"*

"Yes," Bjørn answers, *"that sounds like a good plan."*

As promised, 20 minutes later she is back, bringing her senior colleague. The older colleague looks at the three of us and nods swiftly. Enough of a greeting, as we already have "our" doctor.

They get Bjørn up from the bed but can't make him stand or walk. They examine him a bit more, talk shortly to each other, and conclude they need to consult the consultant as well. It's just that she is in the OR right now. They will be back.

We look at each other. We're a bit exhausted but feel strangely safe. It is as if this Doctor Anna has taken care of all three of us in a very comforting way. It takes another 15 minutes, then she is back:

"Listen—we have looked at the x-rays, and we have even talked to a specialist at the university hospital. It's difficult to say what's wrong. We can see a change in your hip bone, but it's not a normal fracture. That is—if you had been 86 and not 16, a fracture could look like this. Also, the fact that you can't walk strongly indicates something's wrong. I am sorry I don't have a better answer, but it's my first week here, and I'm not into everything yet.

"What we'll do is that we'll take a CT scan now, tonight, and we'll look at the images at tomorrow's morning meeting and then we'll call

you. That is—it might be the doctors from the university hospital who call you instead. So, take a CT scan, go home, and you'll know more tomorrow—does that sound OK?"

"Yes—Thank you."

And so, we did, and all three of us concluded that it felt kind of odd that the information about Doctor Anna only having worked there for a week had not affected our trust in her at all or the feeling of being both seen and comforted.

After Bjørn had fallen to sleep, Christina and I looked at each other and realized we were thinking the same thing—*"We can see a change in your bone—we'll have to discuss this and call you tomorrow"* is something doctors say when they find something really not good on call but have to be sure before breaking the bad news. We had been working long enough as doctors ourselves to know that, sometimes, bone cancer is discovered when looking for fractures.

> We didn't sleep all that well that night, and at 2 p.m. my phone rang—it was Bjørn. *"Dad—help me—I just sneezed and now everything hurts!"*

★ ★ ★

The morning after, I carried my son up the stairs so that he could pee. And then—we waited for the hospital to call.

> Six hours later still no call, so I called them. The ones who had worked yesterday were off now, except for the consultant who was still on duty. *"Hi,"* I said, *"I didn't meet you yesterday, but I understand you were involved in the discussion of my son's x-ray of the hip—do you recall any conclusion from today?"* *"Yes, I do. Didn't they call you?"*
>
> My heart sunk, then skipped a beat, before she continued: *"It was a solid fracture, with many small fragments, yet everything is more or less held in place, so this will heal by itself within 6 weeks."*
>
> *"OK?"*

"Yes. It'll hurt for a week or two, then he can walk as normal. He shouldn't risk falling on it, train too hard, or risk tough physical contact, but as long as he avoids football, skiing, and martial arts for a month and a half he'll be fine."

"OK. Thanks for your time."

"No problem—best of luck now!"

What a roller coaster of emotions, and it hadn't been 24 hours yet since I got the text: *"I'm in the ER!"* So—a fracture, but no surgery. And most of all—no cancer. And still a relief that his face wasn't smashed in the fall. He wasn't so happy himself, although daily taxis to school and a keycard to the elevators were small compensations. His mum and I, however, were simply happy this was a six-week story and not something more.

Not even 24 hours, and an emotional turning point. However, that fulcrum, on which everything seemed to turn happened *before* the results of the CT scan—in the end, making this a story of resolution and healing, rather than a merely painful one of fracture, anguish, and humiliation. It was something that our Doctor Anna did, something that *healed* us, or at least helped to. Exactly what was it? It felt like kindness. What we have come to call *empathy,* perhaps. Had she been a bit older and more experienced, I would have been prone to call it wisdom. But what I do know is that it helped, and that it was what we needed.

Being a teacher of person-centred medicine myself, it was easy to see that Doctor Anna was made of the right stuff and did something right. And I got to tell her just before we left the hospital how happy we were with the way she had welcomed, seen, and treated us. Knowing it in theory, however, is one thing. The *feeling* of being welcomed and comforted and met and seen—that's something else. That counts as *evidence.* That elusive *right* way, the better way, of doing things. Seeing Bjørn opening up, feeling secure, accepting the physical examination, regaining his normal complexion—physically *and* emotionally, though still in pain— something intangible was suddenly made explicit to me—it was there, in plain sight. Something that I try to teach my students. Something that they, and I, all of us, struggle with. Something that is both true and important.

Can this be taught in medical school—or does it all depend on personality traits: Innate virtues over which we have no control? I don't know if anyone knows for certain, but surely, it's worth investing in. Not least, all students who already possess these abilities need to learn not to hide them and that they are part of what makes them good professionals in the end.

9

Dialogue and Healing

John Launer

Introduction

We all become the doctors we are in parallel with becoming the people we are, so I begin with a version of my own story. I'm the son of Jewish refugee parents who arrived in Britain just before the beginning of the Second World War. In the few years that followed, countless numbers of their relatives and school friends in Vienna and Prague were murdered by the Nazis, but in my childhood my parents never spoke about this. They used euphemisms like "it was only cousins that we lost." (This wasn't true, since closer relatives were murdered too, as well as dozens of those who were "only" cousins.) I've spent much of my life gradually unpacking the facts of what happened to these lost individuals and the emotional impact on myself of the surrounding silence. History is full of ironic cycles, and when Britain left the European Union, I felt obliged to claim an Austrian passport in addition to my UK passport, mainly to preserve the right of my children to live and work in continental Europe. At a gathering of our "Right Stuff" group in Rosendal, I showed the newly acquired document to the group in an exercise to share "objects of significance."

My first degree wasn't in medicine but in English literature. My parents had raised me to be more British than the British. I idolized my English teacher at school whose own parents were an earl and a Jewish heiress and who was a devotee of Kleinian psychoanalysis. At university, I was miserable and went into therapy for the first time to try and fathom a concatenation of confusions centred on my sexuality. Like many people in that situation, I then conceived the notion of becoming a psycho-analyst myself. My therapist put me in touch with a social worker and

DOI: 10.1201/9781003593294-9

analyst called Enid Balint, who advised me that my prospects would be better if I trained in medicine and did psychiatry first. I was barely aware that she and her famous refugee husband Michael, who had died a few months earlier, had created the Balint movement, encouraging GPs to join reflective discussion groups in order to develop their emotional literacy. With no scientific background and precious little aptitude, I followed her advice and found a place on a graduate-entry medicine course. My trajectory from there to being at Roshven over 50 years later has repeated echoes of these early influences.

I never became either a psychiatrist or a psychoanalyst, but I did over the subsequent decades take on a succession of professional identities that you could say were similar. I completed training both as a general practitioner and then as a systemic family therapist. I also became a medical writer and an educator. For much of my career, I've practised a combination of these different roles. I spent 29 years doing general practice in a deprived part of London, overlapping with 17 years as a part-time consultant at the Tavistock Clinic, the training organization where the Balints had originally pioneered their own approach. I've published books and now write a regular column for the *British Medical Journal*. I've taught interactional skills widely across Britain, Europe, North America, and Asia. When I get caught up in self-admiration on account of this, I try to recall the words of one of my treasured mentors: "I'd mistrust anyone in a caring profession who hadn't gone into it primarily to sort out themselves." An attraction of the Rosendal-Roshven group isn't principally that there are gurus with greater claims than mine to fame. It's their willingness to share their weaknesses, both physical and emotional. This is a community of self-confessed wounded healers and of vulnerable readers who are able "to hear stories, whether these are works of literature or everyday talk, through the lens of their own troubles, both immediate and anticipated" (Frank, 2022).

The most stabilizing elements in my life have been my wife Lee (a rabbi and educator) and our girl-boy twins who have become a social worker and a doctor. I've been sustained by a deep and spiritual love for the countryside of Wales where I'm writing these words. I've walked over a thousand miles covering its coastal and inland perimeter on foot. The allure of the scenery, geology, and spirit of Rosendal and Roshven are due significantly to their Welsh resonances. In Rosendal, one of the poems I recited to the group was by the poet and priest Gerard Manley Hopkins about the seminary in North Wales where he trained:

I remember a house where all were good
To me, God knows, deserving no such thing:
Comforting smell breathed at very entering,
Fetched fresh, as I suppose, off some sweet wood.
That cordial air made those kind people a hood
All over, as a bevy of eggs the mothering wing
Will, or mild nights the new morsels of Spring:
Why, it seemed of course; seemed of right it should.
Lovely the woods, waters, meadows, combes, vales,
All the air things wear that build this world of Wales;
Only the inmate does not correspond:
God, lover of souls, swaying considerate scales,
Complete thy creature dear O where it fails,
Being mighty a master, being a father and fond.

("In the Valley of the Elwy" by Gerard Manley Hopkins, c. 1877)

Rosendal and Roshven

There are many reasons for being drawn to Norway, but for native English speakers, one of these is a sense of unexpected familiarity when hearing the language. Norwegian can induce the illusion of being perpetually on the verge of understanding it but having a blockage or other impediment to your hearing that prevents you from doing so. This may be a good starting metaphor for contemplating the nature of "The Right Stuff." Another starting point would be one of my favourite quotations about medicine and the doctor–patient relationship by the American physician, psychiatrist, and ethicist Jay Katz (2002):

> *Even in their most intimate relationships, human beings remain strangers to one another. One can only understand another to a limited extent. But the problem runs even deeper. One can only understand oneself to a limited extent. The latter impediment powerfully reinforces the former, making it even more difficult. Patients are not exempt from this human tragedy. Its pervasive impact on all human encounters contradicts one of the most basic and revered professional dogmas: that doctors can be totally trusted because they act only 'in their patients' best interests'. This dogma only compounds the tragedy by assuming an identity of interests and brushing aside the need to clarify differences in expectations and objectives through conversation.*

I've been invited to Rosendal a few times over the years in order to teach, demonstrate, and talk about the particular approach to training in interactional skills for medical and healthcare that I developed known as "Conversations Inviting Change" (Launer, 2018). I devised this during my years at the Tavistock Clinic, along with a colleague called Caroline Lindsey, who had first been my family therapy tutor there. Paradoxically, we designed it as an explicit alternative to the Balint groups which had been created there. We believed that the reflection on emotions that such groups offered wasn't sufficient for developing the precise listening and speaking skills needed in the hurly-burly of everyday work.

"Conversations Inviting Change," often abbreviated to CIC, draws on the principles, ideas, and skills of narrative medicine, but applies these to real-time professional conversations rather than to the study of written texts. CIC incorporates many skills from family therapy, in particular, the approach known as narrative therapy. Its central tenet is that everyone—whether as patient, client, learner or colleague—can benefit from telling stories about their experiences and being skilfully questioned about these. Those of us who teach CIC regard conversations as "moving texts" where both participants (or several, if in a group) can bring about significant shifts in everyone's understanding and perception by means of attentive listening and respectful, non-directive questioning. This means, for example, that within a medical consultation, both patient and doctor may be transformed by the words that pass between them.

Describing such a dynamic and subtle process on the page can give an impoverished or false impression of what CIC involves. In Roshven I showed, as I often do, a teaching video of myself conducting a consultation with a woman suffering from long-standing facial pain, diagnosed as trigeminal neuralgia. Although the woman, Nikki Jones, is an actor, she also has personal experience of the condition, so her performance is highly authentic. Its main purpose is to demonstrate how it is often possible to elicit more information—medical as well as biographical—by listening to a story rather than taking a more formal history. In the video, I focus from the outset on the patient's family and working context and the personal impact on these of her persistent pain. In doing so, I find out a great deal in passing about her past medical treatment, her current medication, and what she is seeking by visiting yet another doctor.

Although she begins the conversation by saying "I want the pain to stop," the patient turns out later to be more interested in strategies for living alongside the pain. To the surprise of many who view the recording, it becomes apparent within a few minutes that she isn't requesting more opiates or a further specialist referral, although this seems the case at first. CIC often has this effect, with patients and doctors alike shifting their own perspectives when their stories are given time to breathe. The video itself can be viewed online on our CIC website, where it is framed by an interview where I discuss it with an academic GP colleague.

Narrative Practice in Action

Training in CIC is similar in one way to a Balint group in focusing on a single individual live "case" at any time: a narrative brought by a group member about an encounter that is bugging them. The chief difference from Balint groups (although not the only one) is that we then assign another group member to interview them using the techniques of therapeutic dialogue. Two or more group members observe the process or act as commentators during appropriately timed pauses in the conversation. A tutor or coach in each group choreographs these conversations, which are intended to act explicitly as a form of training in narrative inquiry.

Such inquiry includes an exploration of the multiple contexts of the predicament being described, along with its complexities and uncertainties, while balancing compassionate acceptance with sensitive challenge. This isn't role play but "real play" where the volunteer speaks in their own voice and in the here and now and the interviewer offers a stance of non-judgemental curiosity into what has happened, what is happening, and what might emerge in an unknowable future. Our intention is that by experiencing this kind of dialogue both as interviewers and narrators, participants will learn ways of listening and speaking that they can apply across the whole range of their work—clinical, collegial, and educational.

I now lead an organization that includes 20 or 30 other active and accredited trainers of CIC, known as the Association of Narrative Practice in Health Care. Whenever and wherever we teach, we always make sure that such small-group practice is preceded by a "fishbowl" exercise where we demonstrate the approach by conducting an interview with a volunteer participant. I did this both at Rosendal and Roshven, holding conversations each time with Margot de Rijke, a young doctor who described herself as already experiencing burnout in the early part of her career. With Margot's consent, I now summarize our conversations and reflect on the ways they demonstrate the principles and practice of CIC. (I have drawn here on Margot's recollection of the conversation as well as my own. Her writing also appears elsewhere in this book.)

In our first conversation, in Roshven, Margot began by explaining how she had entered her first job with enthusiasm. It was in a nursing home with both short- and long-term patients, some with dementia, but most with some degree of cognitive decline. Working with the short-term patients entailed a lot of meetings with next of kin. Many were exhausted from caring for their relatives over time, with home situations becoming intolerable. (Many of the next of kin were themselves also becoming elderly.) It was clear to Margot that these patients and their relatives would profit immensely from a long-term placement at the nursing home, but there was generally no place for them. This resulted in meetings with angry and frustrated next of kin demanding her opinion and agreement—which she found difficult to give because her loyalty was also to the "system" and the people responsible for placement of these elderly people.

Margot described how it became a tug-of-war between her loyalty to her patients and to the system. The senior doctor at the nursing home appeared to believe that Margot was capable of holding these meetings, perhaps not knowing the degree to which the conversations involved this kind of struggle. In any case, the senior did not involve herself in the preparation of the meetings. Margot, being young and wanting to prove herself capable, did not ask for her help, or at least not with the moral aspects of these encounters.

At the time of our conversation, Margot had completed a six-week period of sick leave caused by burnout. Upon her return to work, there had been no conversation with the senior doctor about her struggles or the cause of her burnout. As she described her predicament, Margot began to cry. I asked if it was all right to continue, even with observers present. She said yes: In spite of the tears, she was finding the conversation helpful because she urgently needed to find a way forward. I asked what form "a way forward" might take, and we spent several minutes exploring this. Continuing to weep, Margot recalled something she'd known before but had forgotten to mention: Although she was not contemplating resignation herself, she knew a physical therapist on the ward who was considering doing so because of the same issue. Margot's interconnected release of emotion and memory seemed to have brought about a narrative shift. Her realization that this was not just a problem of her personal vulnerability but a shared and systemic one made it easier to think about the unthinkable, even if it didn't produce an immediate and clear-cut resolution.

To be honest, as an interviewer I was concerned that I might have overstepped a line by taking her into such heightened emotion. I was also worried that my demonstration of questioning technique may have been too detached and technical, given the enormity of her dilemma and feelings. At one point, I asked Margot if a hug would be helpful and she said yes, so I gave her one. At the end of the conversation, I suggested she might want to go for a walk outside with another colleague to debrief privately on our conversation, which she said she did. After she left, I needed a lot of reassurance from the group that it had been right for me to go so deeply into how doctors can be caught up in becoming the unwilling perpetrators of institutional abuse and at the same time being victims of moral injury as a result. In parallel with this, there was the risk that I might be drawn into a different kind of professional abuse by exposing feelings that she wished to keep to herself.

One of the people observing our conversation took notes of all the questions I made in the course of it. Here they all are, slightly adapted for clarity:

- What do I need to know about your work setting in order to understand the story you're going to tell?
- When you offered to have this conversation with me, you said something I didn't quite understand. You said you were "burned out." Can you unpack that for us?
- If this was to be a helpful conversation for you—where would we be at the end of it?
- What are you feeling now, as we speak of this? (Margot starts to tear up.)
- Is it OK if we stay with these emotions? Please let me know if you'd rather take a break now.
- Would a hug be appropriate?
- What do you think your colleagues see in you that makes them feel you're really up to the job?
- What dilemmas does that create for you?
- What can I do or say here and now that would be helpful?
- Where are you now, compared to where you were when we started this conversation?

These questions are fairly typical for CIC. I want to draw attention to some particular features. They are intentionally parsimonious, both in their number and length. Some of them would commonly be used in other conversational approaches like coaching and counselling, but others less so, especially those that explore contexts or invite "a conversation about the conversation itself." They don't intentionally probe for deep emotion but nor do they ignore it. Most of all, they aim to allow maximum narrative space for the person's own description of what has happened, while indicating an expectation that the narrative description will itself change—perhaps to the surprise of both narrator and interviewer.

A common impression for people who attend CIC workshops or come on courses and watch conversations like this is that at first it all seems very familiar ("it's pretty much what I do in practice") and very easy. Yet at the same time, they are puzzled to see narrative and emotional shifts that are far more rapid and extensive than they are used to in their professional conversations. When we get them to practise the approach in small groups, we give the interviewer in each group a clear set of instructions to follow, which we call the "three golden rules":

- Only ask questions (short, simple, open ones).
- Make sure each question follows on from something the narrator has actually said.
- Withhold advice, suggestions, or interpretations.

When the interviewers try to apply these rules in a disciplined way, they discover to their own discomfort (and sometimes shock) that they are addicted to a whole range of conversational habits or tics that actually impede the narrator's words rather than allowing them free and imaginative rein. These habits include leading questions, stereotypical ones drawn from a long-established but limited repertoire, questions based on prior and unexamined assumptions, or ones that have arisen in their own minds but are disconnected from any of the narrative content they have been listening to (or not). The most difficult thing in the world, it seems, is to prevent one's utterances from interfering with the natural potential of someone else's story to take them to the unknown and unexpected places where they need to go.

From experience, we know that it generally takes at least three separate days of intensive coaching to experience the pervasive nature of these impediments and to take the first step in overcoming them. Our courses for trainers of CIC take place in fortnightly sessions lasting a year. Most participants in them nevertheless often report—to our relief—that they still regard themselves as being only at the beginning of a journey to "unlearn" being on automatic as doctors or healthcare professionals.

There are of course many other skills to acquire in CIC. These include learning how to weave normative medical questions into the conversation as well as narrative ones. They also include knowing when to stop: Storytelling never cured anyone of peritonitis. But the overall response we hear from learners is their amazement at how often they have assumed that the best form of conversation was to "take a history" followed by giving advice, while the most effective one is actually to let a story breathe.

The Personal and the Professional: The Two Converge

I didn't see Margot for a year after our conversation at Rosendal, although we exchanged a few emails as I wanted to check how she was. Then I met her again at Roshven. When I asked for a volunteer for my CIC session, she offered to talk about where she now was in her career, and so I did another piece of supervision with her in a fishbowl in front of the rest of the group.

Here, rather than setting down our conversation in any detail, I want to present it in quite a different form, by writing about the context of our conversation rather than the content. Here are the (redacted) entries in my personal diary from four days I spent with the group at Roshven. I will leave readers to garner what they want from these entries. You may be struck by details of the background to how this book was conceived—with indications of deep affection but also tensions within the group, as well as the narrative of how ideas and feelings developed not just in individuals but through relationships and social interactions. Perhaps you will notice my own preoccupation with encroaching frailty, as I reach my mid-70s, when being a doctor converges increasingly not only with my personhood but with being a patient too.

> *Monday 29 May.* We came up yesterday in a seven-seater driven by Edvin with stops for lunch and then a walk in Glencoe. Edvin set us a task for the journey to talk about our identities as doctors—I did so with Edvin in the car and then Caroline on the walk. Edvin told us we had to have breakfast next day at 7, start at 8, have presentations till supper at 8 p.m. and so on, but with no information about breaks. I slept well and we started later than threatened. Iona sensibly challenged Edvin over the timetable. It's good to have Iona here and also Don. I'm

feeling immensely fond of Margot who has agreed to be my supervisee again tomorrow in a fishbowl demonstration of CIC. I've taken some opportunities to take time out and snooze or catch up on other work including preparation for teaching in Japan in July. The beauty of this place on a sea loch and the excellence of the food (cooked by Peter's son Jack) are the main attractions. I miss Tom Hutchinson and his mischief from last year in Rosendal. The ethnic and professional homogeneity is also striking.

Tuesday 30 May. I'm preoccupied with the possibility of having a bladder infection and what that might mean for the rest of this week, but more importantly for Japan. Low back discomfort this morning, possibly from the bed, but also feeling the cold. It may all mean nothing, but I told Peter early this evening: He's going to Edinburgh tomorrow and will come back on Thursday with dipsticks and antibiotics. Otherwise, the highlight of the day was a very good morning session on CIC. I showed a demonstration video of a consultation, to a very good response. I supervised Margot as a follow-up to last year (she cried again but reported she has found it cathartic both times). Later on, we had sessions from Iona on the overuse of diagnostic terms, Don and Edvin on phronesis, and Ron Epstein on appreciative inquiry. I paired off with Victoria who is recovering from possible COVID, but we then had a nice conversation about awkward moments (I talked about a poor demonstration of CIC I carried out in Wales last month). I polished off some work stuff including invoices, went to supper in the other house, a delicious paella, but left at 10 during the music.

Wednesday 31 May. Our last official day at Roshven although I'm staying on a couple of days. My prostate is annoying but tolerable, and I'll probably just need to live with it through Japan. I talked to Ron and Edvin who both found drugs for prostatism somewhat useful but not totally. A good morning of presentations and workshops, and we're starting to plan the book. I did a short session on the three golden rules (asking everyone to focus on a "journey of discovery" they had made). I got very sleepy afterwards and dozed off. Half the group left, including Don and Iona. I slept for two hours then did some writing. Supper for the remaining seven of us, then we all walked down to the beach and then stood around the fire pit, but the midges defeated us.

Thursday 1 June. The best moment of the day was discovering from dipsticks (brought by Peter from Edinburgh) that I do have a bladder infection. Shocked to find I also have sugar in my urine, but Peter thinks this is probably due to being on dapagliflozin for my heart. The glycosuria was at first far more of a shock than the infection, but I'll stop the dapagliflozin as well as taking the antibiotics and see what happens. It's very reassuring to be among doctors and to develop a plan through talking to them. I snoozed a couple of times during the day but felt better doing so after the diagnosis. A mellow evening at the other house with a fish stew made by Peter and the company of his wife Deborah and Jack's partner Hannah. I told jokes, including Jewish ones; listened to music; watched the sunset; and hugged Lizzie who is leaving first thing tomorrow. A good ending all round.

★   ★   ★

Reading these extracts, you may be disappointed that Margot couldn't report that our dramatic conversation the previous year had led to a miraculous transformation in her approach to her career. But such a transformation isn't something I would necessarily have expected, even though it does sometimes happen. At their heart, CIC and "The Right Stuff" are about something else: evolving conversations that avoid offering quick fixes or the illusion of definitive solutions, but instead nurture and support people as they navigate through their own vulnerable lives.

Conclusion

A year later, Peter and I had a conversation over the kitchen table at his house in Edinburgh. I was sceptical about whether our proposed book would work out or even be completed. Peter, by contrast, spoke passionately about the nature of "The Right Stuff." Here is an abridged version of how he summarized it to me in writing afterwards:

We are all alone, mortal, vulnerable subjects. The recognition of this predicament—our limited lives, the prospect of the loss and the end of everything, gives us suffering. It also gives us value. Suffering is always, entirely, subjective—private and ultimately un-knowable to any but its subject. The purpose of medicine is the recognition and mitigation of the other's suffering. Medicine has lately become an increasingly techno-scientific discourse, nested within a particular cultural context—expressions like "late modernity," "late capitalism," get used here. Medicine functions now, increasingly, by reifying suffering—turning it into an objective scientific discourse, whereby it is measured, counted, systemized, cured. In its time and place, that can be incredibly effective! But there is an evident contradiction at the core of this interaction—between what is the irreducibly subjective nature of suffering, and the objectifying, systematizing discourse of medicine. The quality of a subject's suffering reveals itself through narration. Healing must necessarily involve a kind of hermeneutics. Narrativity is the potential bridge between the suffering subject, and the objectifying discourse of medicine. Without the bridge of narrativity, the two discourses can't engage with one another.

But being a narrative, rather than purely analytic discourse, has certain implications. In any clinical space, suffering is always distributed unevenly and unpredictably between healer and patient. The healer is always, also, a suffering subject (Thank God!) and that suffering always influences outcomes. So, the healer needs certain qualities and dispositions in order to be able to function in her role. These might include, amongst many others— practical wisdom, aka phronesis. And a particular presence, which can be cultivated by certain skills—such as a reflective disposition and the practice of eg mindfulness. And habits of self-care and self-management, which are diverse and individual.

And finally, there is something ideological about "The Right Stuff." It is potentially life changing. I can attest to that—I've spoken about how CIC, for example, has changed my practice, in a very practical and pragmatic way. We need to be able to capture some of how we, as a group in Rosendal and Roshven achieved the work that we have done, in order that we might develop and promote this thinking.

I hope that in this chapter I have managed to advance some of the mission Peter laid out.

Ever since I was a medical student, it has been fashionable on and off to praise and promote an approach to medicine known as "biopsychosocial," following the American internist and psychiatrist George Engel, who first proposed the term. I have to confess I've never fallen in love with the name or the idea. It so often seems to imply (whether Engel intended this or not) that the biological, psychological, and social domains can be neatly distinguished from each other and that the physician is an independent observer with the capacity to tease these apart and make authoritative judgements about the interconnections between them. With my personal background, and especially since acquiring an understanding of narrative through family therapy training, I have tended to see such an understanding of medicine as too concrete, too certain, and too positivist in the philosophical sense.

For me, these apparently discrete domains are interfused in people's lives in ways that are fluid, nuanced, and elusive. In a similar fashion—to use the language of the Jewish philosopher Martin Buber—there may be no very clear boundary between the vulnerable "I" in the person of the physician and the suffering "Thou" of the patient or colleague who must somehow be encountered. If we can help students and learners to gain a sense of the precarious and fragile nature of this encounter and of its wondrous potential to sustain and transform us, we will have done our jobs as medical educators.

References

Frank, A. (2022). Why wounded storytellers need to be vulnerable readers. *Narrative Works: Issues, Investigations, and Interventions, 11,* 61–72.

Katz, J. (2002). *The silent world of doctor and patient.* Revised edition. Johns Hopkins Press.

Launer, J. (2018). *Narrative-based practice in health and social care: Conversations inviting change.* Routledge.

10

Attending to the Unsaid: On Knowing, Care, and Voice

Caroline Engen and Edvin Schei

Det er den draumen me ber på at noko vedunderleg skal skje, at det må skje – at tidi skal opna seg, at hjarta skal opna seg, at dører skal opna seg, at berget skal opna seg, at kjeldor skal springa – at draumen skal opna seg, at me ei morgonstund skal glida inn på ein våg me ikkje har visst um.	It's that dream we carry that something wonderful will happen, that it must happen – that time will open, that hearts will open, that doors will open, that the mountain will open, that springs will gush forth – that the dream will open, that one morning we will glide into a harbor we didn't know was there.
Olav H. Hauge	Robert Bly's translation

Poem by Olav H. Hauge reproduced with permission from Samlaget

Late May. Four days, each stretching longer toward midsummer. A Scottish landscape—the sea, the sun. Two cabins by the water, set apart yet open to the world. Thirteen physicians—thirteen people—gathered. Drawn together, not by a single answer, but by a shared question: *What Is the Right Stuff of Medicine?*

DOI: 10.1201/9781003593294-10

For many, the more seasoned physicians in the group, this question has been a lifelong companion—woven into decades of practising, teaching, living. They have tried to answer it—if only tentatively—through the ways they have worked, the choices they have made, the spaces they have carved out for something different. For others, still in their first years of physicianship, the question has been forced into articulation—actualized—more harshly, when limits of medicine, or of themselves within it, suddenly became undeniable.

What Is the Right Stuff of Medicine? A question shaped by absence, by lack, by all that is missing, all that no longer holds. Therefore, not only a question but also a longing for something different—a manifestation of hope. And with this question a flow of other questions: What is it about our experiences as doctors that brings us together? That has made the lot of us uneasy, critical, deviant even—across different ages, countries, specialties, perspectives? What does this uneasiness reveal—not just about medicine but about ourselves within it? What does this uneasiness reveal about *the right stuff of medicine*?

To us, these are not abstract questions. They are concerns—matters of care, pressing and unresolved.

Among the thirteen were four hosts. Through a year of planning, we had imagined, reflected, and theorized how to explore these questions (see Chapter 17). Together we had carefully crafted a frame from which we hoped a space would emerge—a space where the question *What Is the Right Stuff of Medicine?* could be opened, explored, and held at the same time.

Now—anticipation, expectation, a flicker of fear. Hosting is never neutral. To open and hold a space, to invite others into it—is to step into the unknown. This chapter is about some of what emerged, some of what we learned, some of what we came to know. It is about an experiment and an experience—of holding space for disruption, for silence, for voice. It is about presence, listening, being with. About knowing more than we can say. Of what it takes to care. It is about what some of us are coming to understand as strands of *The Right Stuff of Medicine*.

Through this, two of the hosts' voices weave together—reflecting and navigating—moving between theorizing and experiencing, questioning and sensing, holding and disrupting, receiving and being received.

Edvin: Medicine is interwoven with all that is human. Does medicine in its current formats connect with all that is human? Or has it become increasingly distanced from the very lives it seeks to heal and the lives of those whose task it is to heal—their relationship fragmented by specialization, constrained by bureaucracy, driven by compliance rather than presence? Perhaps medicine itself is not immune to injury; perhaps it, too, is in need of healing. Of being tended to, questioned, and cared for as not just as a system, but as a shared practice that holds the weight of our collective vulnerabilities and responsibilities.

Caroline: Physicians have long been stewards of health, but what does it mean to steward medicine itself? Not only to ask what is worth preserving, what is worth transforming—but to hold open the questions of *How medicine fails—how we fail?* To recognize medicine not as something fixed, but as something in need of care. To ask: *What is at stake? What must be accounted for? What does it take to be accountable? What am I responsible for?*

To me the question, *What Is the Right Stuff of Medicine?* is not just a matter of knowing, but of what is at stake in knowing. To ask this question is to recognize that medicine is not self-evident, that its forms and functions are neither fixed nor neutral. It is to acknowledge that what counts as legitimate knowledge, what is valued, preserved, or discarded, is always also shaped by forces beyond the clinic. To ask this question is to recognize that the question matters. There is something at stake. To ask this question is also to ask: *What is required of us to provide even a tentative answer?*

Edvin: Medicine, as it is often practised, is structured around the imperative to do, to decide, to act. But what if good doctoring also requires other approaches? Different kinds of attention? Other ways of knowing?

How can we identify and make relevant that which medical education, institutionalized medical practice, public expectation, and tradition might be blind to and tend to make us blind to? And how can four days of dialogues and interaction create enough change to point us in meaningful directions? Nurture enough strength to act?

Caroline: We know more than we say. We know more than we can say. We know more than can be said. We know more than can be recognized.

Knowing is shaped by boundaries—of thought, of who is granted authority as a knower, of language, of what is visible, audible, and decipherable. But invisibility is not absence. Just because something is hidden doesn't mean it isn't there. It lives in us, in what we carry, in the ways we move, listen, and care. In the ways we fail. The challenge is to bring forward what is obscured—and more so, to trust it, to trust ourselves, and to let it shape how we practice, how we live, how we commune.

Edvin: We know more than we say—insight is sometimes felt before it is named, sensed before it is spoken. Collectively, we might be able to find words, and thereby strength.

Lebanese poet Kahlil Gibran wrote: "Your hearts know in silence the secrets of the days and the nights. But your ears thirst for the sound of your heart's knowledge. You would know in words that which you have always known in thought. You would touch with your fingers the naked body of your dreams. And it is well that you should" (Gibran, 1923).

Caroline: The Hungarian-British polymath Michael Polanyi, who also trained as a physician, says, "we can know more than we can tell" (Polanyi, 1966). But often, we don't trust what we know in our bodies. As physicians we've been taught that real knowledge must be measured, calculated, proven. Yet we know much more—knowledge that works through our hands, our gestures, our posture; in the silences we keep; in the unease that lingers when numbers look fine but something still feels off; in the subtle shift of someone's breath; in the space between words—when what is spoken does not quite hold, when someone insists they are fine, but the weight of the moment reveals otherwise.

To practise with a richer awareness is to honour this knowing. It is to trust that lived experience is knowledge, too. Not separate from theory, but woven into it. Not something to prove, but something to hold. Because knowing isn't just about words. It's about presence. It's about care.

Edvin: Not only do we know more than we can tell, as Polanyi observed. We also tell more than we can know. Humans tend to immensely overestimate their ability to understand, explain, and decide their own behaviour (Nisbett & Wilson, 1977). Each of us can easily see that people around us are living out values and worldviews that stem not from themselves, but from the powers around them. Yet we tend to believe that we do not suffer from the same tendency. This is captured in the Book of Matthew: "Why do you look at the speck of sawdust in your brother's eye and pay no attention to the plank in your own eye?"

Knowing this, we must be self-critical. But not so humble as to be impotent. As philosopher Bertrand Russel observed, "The trouble with the world is that the stupid are cocksure and the intelligent are full of doubt." How do we find the soft spot of wisdom—the balance between arrogance and self-effacement?

Caroline: To know differently, to know more, we must disrupt: Disrupt the style of thought, disrupt the assumptions and hierarchies of the collective, disrupt language, disrupt the very conditions of intelligibility and legibility.

Disrupt—not to destroy or abandon, but to create something different—a space for thinking, for creativity, for co-production. I see disruption as an opening, a way of using contrast and surprise to make the taken-for-granted visible, unsettled, and available for questioning. Disruption as a means of creating a space where coming to know is not about repeating or exchanging what has already been thought, but about thinking together, making room for the unexpected—for something else to emerge. For what remains unspoken, for what is rendered unspeakable, for what resists articulation, for what remains illegible.

Edvin: In preparation for the second seminar, each person was asked to bring an artefact—a token that signalled or represented what gave them strength, carrying capacity as professionals, as persons. Something that had, in one way or another, made the question *What Is the Right Stuff of Medicine?* stand out to them—made the question both possible to hold and impossible to ignore.

On the first evening of our seminar, they shared their artefacts with the group, offering reflections on strength and how they sustained it. After the round of sharing, each participant was asked to prepare, over the next days, a space for the others to step into—an invitation into a practice that foregrounded something that embodied or revealed what strength meant to them—what strength felt like to them.

For each person, each space, and each practice exchanged, a small coloured stone marble would be collected in a jar. By the end of the seminar, each of us would have a small jar containing thirteen soft, polished, heavy spheres—each representing a person, an experience, and a practice—a jar of strength.

Over the following days, workshops and plenary discussions unfolded, interwoven with these spaces—moments of immersion, invitations into another's way of holding strength. A backdrop to dialogue, a counterpoint to discourse, a disruption of the usual flow of knowledge. Each practice, each offering, part of a collective rhythm—one that made space not just for what was already known but for what was still taking shape.

Caroline: I sit cross-legged on a yoga mat, my back to the window. Behind me, the ocean mirrors the rising sun. A space where everything is still possible, where everything is still uncertain.

This was what I had insisted on, argued for, almost pleaded for—spaces in the seminar where we wouldn't just talk about being, but be. *Being sessions.* Not a break, not a pause from the important work, but the very core of it. Supportive, yet disruptive. A web meant to weave through the seminar, to hold it, to challenge it.

Met with scepticism, with resistance, with unease. A risky project. Disruptive—potentially destructive? Tension within me, my own unease. Why was this so important to me? Why was I willing to stand by it, despite the discomfort?

How would it be received? How would I be received?

The marbles sitting with me, all of them. Still. Unmoved. Small and solid, yet impossibly heavy—the weight of possible failure, of complete rejection. The quiet fear that what I had fought for would be dismissed. That I would be dismissed.

Breath expands, retracts. Present. Holding the space as they enter, filling the room. Holding the discomfort.

I invite them to settle, to breathe, to join in shared presence. I encourage them to lie down, close their eyes if it feels right. To listen. To receive the sounds—the ocean, a Tibetan gong, Koshi chimes.

I move between them, playing.

The deep roars and vibrating weight of the gong resonate through flesh, setting it in motion. The delicate, shimmering tones of the chimes brush lightly against silence, drifting above, almost caressing the skin.

I leave them in silence.

Then, I bring them back.

I invite them to notice—not just the sound, but the sensation. Not just what they hear, but what shifts. Hold that awareness. Then, write. Not to analyse, not to explain. Just to capture. Felt. Embodied. Immediate.

What they make of it—I don't know. But they make something.

Edvin: As Caroline asks us to lie down on the floor, there is hesitation in the room. Glances are exchanged. It's our first hours together, we don't know each other. What is this? For a minute, I am as much aware of the fidgeting of people around me as I am of the droning tinkling sounds that vibrate through my body. As the others become quiet, I slowly relax. Breathing, I allow the sound to engulf me. I try to stay focused, but cannot keep my thoughts from wandering, returning again and again to the strangeness of what we are doing and why it seems to be so important. The sounds recede from my awareness as thoughts take over. A stream of consciousness. A stream of fragmented thought—on the people in the room, their presence, their distance. Who are they? What have they carried here? The quiet weight of their bodies on the floor, the uneven rhythm of breath, the way hesitation lingers before surrender.

On self—the pull between immersion and observation. The mind resists stillness, resists silence, clinging to thought, to movement, to the need to make sense. Should I let go? Or should I hold on?

On thought itself, how it intrudes—uninvited, relentless. How it demands attention, disrupts presence, keeps reaching for explanation, for structure. What am I supposed to be thinking? Am I supposed to be thinking at all?

On exposure—how silence makes things visible, how stillness makes things louder. Thought unfiltered, self unguarded. Nowhere to hide from what rises to the surface.

A stream of hesitation, of resistance, of fragile openness.

As the gongs drone on, I continue to breathe slowly. My eyes are closed. I sense other bodies breathing the same air, accepting the same sound.

A final thought—if the goal is to catalyse thinking, we must somehow create trust.

Caroline: The first time I attended a sound bath, I was struck by my own resistance—fighting back against the intrusion of sound, overwhelmed not by the intensity, but how it moved through me. It wasn't demanding anything from me, the gong, only offering something for me—and that, somehow, was the hardest to accept—to receive. That resistance became a focal point of meditation for me, a theme I would return to time and time again—resurfacing in clinical, collegial, and personal encounters. When a colleague would look at me in a way that made me feel seen—too seen—at moments when I wanted to hold myself together. When I realized I was deflecting gestures of kindness, of recognition, of care, because it felt easier to keep moving than to receive it.

I saw it in others too—in the way students stiffened when I asked them to reflect rather than recite, as if the invitation itself was too exposing. In the way some patients met my compassion with scepticism, testing whether it was safe to trust. In the way care itself could feel intrusive—too much, too close.

It became for me a meditation on what it means to be truly open and receptive—of what is required, of what is at stake. A meditation on why that matters in medicine. A meditation on why it matters to me. A meditation on how resistance wasn't always refusal. Sometimes, it was a shield. A way of holding onto what felt safe, what felt known.

In this seminar we wanted to create a space for generative thought—for co-production, where knowledge is not just exchanged but emergent. And thinking anew is rarely comfortable; it demands unlearning, a willingness to sit with discomfort, to let old certainties loosen their grip. It is easier to defend what we already know than to risk the vulnerability of thinking together—to allow ideas to be unsettled, reshaped, even undone. But without that risk, without that opening, nothing new can emerge.

Now, I wanted to invite my colleagues into that dialogue of tension—not in an abstract, detached, or theoretical way, but embodied. Because, if the goal is to catalyse thinking, beyond trust, we must somehow create and sustain openness.

As such, my small gong bath was an experience within a larger experience of exchange—an invitation to give and receive, not in any particular way, but mindfully. To reflect on what it brought forward, how it felt. To notice resistance, openness, and the quiet shifts in between.

And as the sound of the chimes faded, the first marbles found their way—one of the same kind into thirteen small jars. An offering of something shared but not yet fully understood.

Edvin: To become a doctor you have to learn to think, talk, and act in certain ways. Those ways are prescribed by medical school's lectures, exams, and the "hidden curriculum," the norms of professionalism that a newcomer will glean from what physicians, older students, and other role models say, who they talk to, how they talk, what they laugh at, what makes them roll their eyes, who they admire, who they despise (Hafferty, 2016). Equipped for adaptation and survival, humans have deeply automated, non-conscious skills for picking up and copying the subtle clues of power and weakness, shame and pride, that increase or decrease social standing (Bargh & Chartrand, 1999; Hayles, 2014). Learning to become a doctor is not only, and perhaps not foremost, to learn medical facts and skills, but to learn the clinical gaze (Foucault, 1975)—a way of seeing, feeling, and reacting to disease, sick people, and suffering that aligns with what is normal and taken for granted in physicians' community of practice (Good, 1994; Wenger, 1998).

Caroline: We know more than we *can* say. What is sayable is shaped by norms, by unwritten rules of decorum and authority—by who is permitted to speak and what kinds of knowledge are granted legitimacy. Knowing is never neutral—it is shaped, structured, constrained. Ludwik Fleck, himself a physician, reminds us that thought does not emerge in isolation; it is formed within thought collectives, *Denkkollektive*. Medical training is not just about acquiring knowledge but about being brought into communion—being inducted into a particular thought style, a way of perceiving, reasoning, and making sense of the world that, in sum, defines the very boundaries of what can be known, said, and acted upon. It shapes not only what is considered evidence but also what remains imperceptible, what is dismissed, and what is rendered unthinkable (Fleck, 1979). To break free from these constraints takes more than knowledge; it takes courage. The courage to resist, to think beyond inherited frames. But also the courage to let go—to recognize when structure is necessary and when it must be loosened, unmade.

Coloured marbles, exchanged in silence, accumulating in a jar. A simple act, yet one that breaks with the expected flow, foregrounding what typically remains backgrounded—context, hierarchies, structures of practice that shape what can be said, what can be known, and what remains unspoken. A way of calling attention to the unnoticed—to how knowledge circulates, to who speaks and who remains silent, to the ways medicine disciplines attention and obscures its own conditions of intelligibility.

Edvin: Danish philosopher Søren Kierkegaard is paraphrased as saying "To dare is to lose one's footing momentarily. Not to dare is to lose oneself." For me, a jolt that makes me lose my footing, unpleasant though it might be, can make me aware that what I know is but a fragment of what there is to know. It can make me aware that what I take to be *understanding* is my self-made tapestry, woven of prejudice and assumptions, patterns of interpretation that, like the algorithms on the internet, force upon me perceptions of everything, of who those others are and who I am to them, as a person or as a doctor. As I get to know the workings of my mind, I realize that I need correction, guidance, adjustments, that I must welcome uncertainty and fallibility to live well (Schei et al., 2019).

Thinking is an array of activities, more than, but including, the calculations of the analytic mind, of the chess player or the physicist. To think is to ask questions with a beginner's mind, to see the strangeness of well-known worlds, and sometimes realize in a glimpse that the alien is also familiar. Thinking is reality-making. By creating growth, power, and agency, thinking can be akin to healing. If I understand better, if I am more mindful of how stories, biases, and deeply automated impulses constitute all human beings, myself included, I will be less constrained by those patterns. I will be less afraid of being honest, less lonely, less prone to alienation and suffering.

Real thinking is not to rehearse old thoughts. Real thinking stems from messy attempts to grasp a yet nebulous meaning, it is fumblingly to try words, tell stories, hold emotions, seek guidance. Thinking is to exercise and reveal one's character while leaping into unknowns. It is to dare, it is often joyful, it can be strengthening. Thinking is to be unprotected, it can happen when I am porous, receptive to impressions, moods, mirroring, open to strange ideas about the world, about others, about myself and who I am for them. When I am open and porous, I am vulnerable, out of control. One cannot really think without being at risk.

Caroline: Coloured marbles, exchanged in silence, accumulating in a jar. Not rupture, not destruction, but a shift that makes visible what is usually overlooked. The weight of a marble in the palm, the pause it demands, the space it creates. Not merely an interruption, but an opening—a moment where something else might surface.

Edvin: Lying down with strangers, under a shower of sound from gongs and bells gently hammered by this enigmatic colleague, takes courage. To surrender, be held, relinquish control. It takes courage to trust, courage to be open. The potential for shame is ever-present where people come together. The prospect of shame holds us in place. To avoid it we seek stability, control, predictability, recognition. Not the best recipe for change, curiosity, or discovery.

I had brought an old framed black and white photo to circulate in the group of colleagues. It portrayed a young thin man playing the mandolin while his two-year-old son affectionately hangs around his neck. The boy looks at the photographer, presumably his mother. I am the little boy; my father is the mandolin player.

I was 13 when the following happened; it must have been the early 1970s. He worked as a GP in a small Norwegian town on the west coast. Every afternoon he returned to the old farm tucked away in the forest where we lived. That was a place for cutting trees and making firewood, caring for vegetables and fruit trees, moving heavy rocks in the wheelbarrow to build walls. In the afternoons, he loved this kind of work. After a while he would sit down comfortably in the dirty wheelbarrow that snugly fit his big belly, take off his gloves, light a cigarette, and ask me to fetch a beer in the cellar.

One day as he sat there in his work clothes, enjoying the smoke and the sounds of summer, a guest arrived. It was the local teacher, a rather stern handsome man in his 30s, well-known as a leading figure in the pietist prayer house environment that still held great power in those days. One would never voice critical or divergent opinions to people in these circles or openly drink alcohol, mention sex, make jokes about religion, or use even the mildest swear word in front of a devout Christian. Conformity was the rule.

My father had spent years of his childhood in hospital, with osteomyelitis in a fractured femur after falling from an apple tree in the neighbour's garden when he was six. He couldn't get out of bed and was cared for by nuns who in the name of God had confined the boy to endless boredom, even denying him access to the radio, except for daily Mass. The experience gave my father the dream of becoming a doctor, and it eradicated his faith in God as well as his appetite for rule-following and conformity.

The teacher wanted to discuss some trouble at school with the doctor. My father had the habit of spicing up his language when he became engaged, and the same happened then, as he spoke from his wheelbarrow to the tall teacher standing in front of him. The teacher frowned and said, "I must ask you not to swear in front of me." My father took a deep puff of the cigarette, as if collecting his mind. Then, meeting the teacher's eyes, he said the memorable words: "I bloody well swear as much as it suits me, when I sit in my own wheelbarrow."

It is the audacity to be slightly crazy, to risk holding one's own even at considerable social cost, that I associate with my father at his best. I call it Wheelbarrow Power. I think of it when I see the picture of the young man concentrating on the mandolin, little Edvin over his shoulder, their warm bodies close together, total trust, the boy looking up as if on behalf of both of them, saying with his eyes "my father and I, we are the same stuff." Independence grows from attachment.

I need my Wheelbarrow Power in situations where I feel under pressure, not taken seriously, pushed around by people with power. In such discussions I have felt ill at ease, alone, afraid of humiliation above all. It is tempting to crumble, to go along with what they say, get a pat on the shoulder, belong. I often succumb. But not always. Sometimes I find my Wheelbarrow Power and say what I believe to be true.

I have wondered whether it is at all wise to speak one's mind in such situations. Sometimes it feels like self-harm, of no practical use, the world remains the same and I am further outside it. But I reckon my acts change me. Virtues are learned through virtuous action, said Aristotle. Wheelbarrow Power increases with use.

Caroline: As Edvin talked about courage—the image of his father, cigarette in hand, sitting in a wheelbarrow—my thoughts drifted to my own father. His anger at God, who he felt had abandoned him. His anger at late modernity, at its fragmentation. Yet his never-ending curiosity, his relentless need to make sense of his condition—of *our* condition—always a new book in hand. His yellowed fingers from a lifetime of smoking. The trace of whiskey on his breath. His pain, his stamina, his stubbornness, his hopefulness. His death.

How courage, integrity, and destruction live so close together. How hard it is to pull them apart, to name one without the other. What does it mean to be courageous? To resist, to disrupt, to refuse? When is silence strength, and when is it fear? When is speaking up a necessity, and when is it just defiance dressed as principle? I used to think courage was about standing firm, about speaking up. Now, I wonder if it's just as much about knowing when to let go, knowing when to let be—not in isolation, but in communion. That was my father's plea—not to intrude, not to judge, not to change, but to take a share in the weight of existence, in the unspoken burdens we carry—in the unspoken strength with which we carry—in the quiet dignity of simply being alongside one another.

Edvin: Pride, shame, identification, and conformity are unavoidable elements of becoming fully human. Using a computer metaphor, socialization is akin to the installation of millions of programs and algorithms, the software needed to function as a person. But it comes with a risk, namely that the person becomes too much of a machine-like executor of the programs he or she happens to have internalized. How can we move beyond that level? How can we become our own "computer programmers," not just operated by our capabilities and past experiences, but operators who can use those resources, and seek out new ones, to understand, create, and act?

This is the level of self-awareness, of discovering our resources and vulnerabilities, of exploring self and others in dialogue, of reflection-on-action and reflection-in-action (Schei et al., 2019). For professionals, this level of functioning is attainable through experience, with others, in an approach to knowledge that the Greek philosophers called *praxis*.

Praxis is what people do when they take into account all the circumstances and exigencies that confront them at a particular moment and then, taking the broadest view they can of what it is best to do, they act. . . . It may be a moment when it is time to speak out. It may be a moment when the most important thing to do is to show care. It may be a moment when one must listen. It may be a moment when it is necessary to tell the patient that his illness is terminal, or the student that he must leave the room.

(Kemmis, 2012, p. 150)

How do I know that I take "the broadest view" of what is best to do? I cannot know. I can only try to engage with and be true to the entirety of my lived experience, also that which seems to fall outside or contradict conventional wisdom. But I need help to do that—to find the courage to face shame, the honesty to question my understanding, and the voice to craft my thoughts. The voice to howl, if need be.

Caroline: We know more than can be recognized. The jar, slowly filling—not just with the tangible weight of marbles but with something harder to name: Gestures of recognition, fragments of strength, ways of knowing that had been offered and received, some barely noticed, some quietly set aside, some slipping into silence.

Each stone, for me, a marker of what I could receive and what I could not—of profound appreciation, bewilderment, uncertainty, resistance.

Marbles of embodied and intellectual curiosity, marbles of disembodiment—word games, thought games, playing with perspectives—shifting focus—narrowing in, expanding out.

The sun is setting, casting long shadows. A slow dance, not for anyone, not for anything, just movement in response to the air cooling against my skin, the weight of the day falling away. A moment entirely my own—not performing, not proving, just being.

Marbles of courage, of emotional honesty and vulnerability.

Holding the gaze of someone I barely know. Telling them they are good enough. Hearing them tell me the same. A hesitation, a lingering.

Thoughts of my patients. How I doctor. My children. How I parent. My husband. How I partner. What I say, what I model. Tensions, imperfections. The weight of care. Am I really enough?

Marbles of trust—that one is enough, yet not too much.

A gathering, voices filling the room. The expectation of singing. A tightening in my chest—hesitation. The feeling of not quite belonging, of not speaking the same language. The quiet effort to match a rhythm I do not entirely understand. The tension of wanting to be part of it, yet fearing the weight of my own voice within the collective sound. Then, across the room, a glance—recognition. A fellow hesitancy, a shared uncertainty. Connection, not through confidence, but through the quiet trust that we are here, and that is enough.

Marbles of care—not as intrusion, but as responsiveness.

Later, he sings. His voice fills the room—unsteady at first, then gathering strength, reaching further. A presence unfolding, vulnerability carried not as weakness but as something else— something expansive, something generous. The warmth in the room shifts—not just listening, but holding space. Not expecting, not demanding, simply allowing. I feel it settle in me—the quiet power of witnessing someone step into their own voice. A moment not about confidence, but about offering something real, unguarded. A reminder that strength is not the absence of hesitation but the courage to stay with it.

Marbles of reception—not as passive acceptance, but as openness.

I sit in that space, unexpectedly moved, unexpectedly grateful. Inspired—not by certainty, but by the trust it takes to be seen. The quiet courage of offering something unfinished, something raw. The way a moment can expand—not by force, but by allowing. To receive is not to take, not to claim, but to make room. To let something emerge without rushing to define or resolve. To recognize that presence—simply being here, neither too much nor too little—is enough.

Marbles of silence, calm, and connection.

Sitting in a canoe, the water so still it barely registers movement. The paddle rests across my lap, forgotten for a moment. Beside me, another presence—neither intrusive nor distant, just there. The silence here is different—not absence, but something more alive. A shared quiet that asks for nothing. The weight of solitude, but not loneliness.

Marbles of release.

Edvin: "When I feel miserable, exhausted, disappointed with myself and useless as a doctor, I have discovered that the bad weather of Scotland can be really helpful." Lara, who is originally Dutch, smiles wryly. "I go out bareheaded and let the rain fall in my face. Or I walk along a beach and let the wind ruffle my hair." There are nods and hums of recognition in the group of people as we hear Lara talking from the chair in front of the big windows, through which we can see trees and cliffs surrounding a little cove. The sky is blue. It is the morning session of the second day. Lara, a family doctor in her 30s, seems hesitant. She looks around, as if trying to guess what is expected of her in this eccentric gathering of unknown doctors, several of whom are a generation older and definitely not hesitant about letting their thoughts be heard. Lara takes a deep breath before she continues. "When I am alone, when the wind is strong or the waves make sounds, I scream. Maybe you think I'm crazy. I haven't talked about it with people. But here. . . . You ask what I do to get through my days, how I create what some of you have called carrying capacity. . . . Well, I sometimes howl and scream at the top of my lungs, and it feels good. As if I make myself aware that I am me, I make my own decisions, I don't have to do only what everybody else does and says. So, my gift to you, the exercise that I invite you to do, is to go out and make sounds. Yell and scream if you like. We'll be back here in twenty minutes. We are not going to talk about it in the plenary afterwards, just make notes in the diaries you've been given, those who want."

Now it is the older group members who look somewhat hesitant, as they slowly get up and step outside.

As Lara announces her being session exercise, my abdomen immediately tightens. A rush of thoughts and voices well up: Do I have to do this? Will I dare to make sounds? Will my sound be nice? What a stupid thought, Edvin, you should be above this, don't be so cowardly. Do you really need to care what they will think? You're so vain! They will have more than enough with their own screaming! But what if I make myself ridiculous? Everybody will hear my sound and judge me! I am a leader here, I don't want to look stupid, I don't want to SOUND stupid! But I cannot NOT scream, I am one of the leaders, I must model the courage, the freedom, the strength to be yourself that we say this seminar is about! Oh shut up now, and get out there!

As I step out in the mild morning air, I see others finding their way towards the beach, the cliffs, the little patches of forest. Not much to hear, only John mutters "scream, scream, scream, scream" with semi-loud voice as he carefully steps on the flagstones toward the little brook from the marshes behind the house. That helps. If he can make sound, I can too. I walk towards a cliff jutting up on the other side of the stony beach. As I scramble up, I make my first shouts. Now I hear other voices in the distance, competing with the soft background sound of the ocean swell, the faint wind, the calls of seagulls. I fill my lungs and make a long, deep sound. Do I sound stupid now? Do they notice? Again this ridiculous inner dialogue. Here I am, supposedly using Lara's guidance to find my own voice, and all I do is try to control how I impress the others. So much for wisdom and maturity!

Again and again, I fill my lungs and howl across the beach, over the gentle waves of the cove, along the deep fjord towards the distant islands on the horizon. I notice that I am getting used to the situation, to using my voice in this ridiculous way, to the others potentially noticing. I almost forget to think about them, though I hear their voices here and there. I observe how my strong voice disappears into nature. When it's time to return to the cabin, I feel a mild regret. The inner voices are quiet now. I notice that I feel neither shame nor pride. I am calm.

I have exposed my naked sound and survived.

I could have stayed here longer, singing to open space.

Caroline: I step into the landscape barefoot. Balancing on sharp stones. Sink down into wet moss, cool against my skin. Firm footing at the coastal rock—ocean reaching toward my toes.

With the sound of a voice piercing the air, I suddenly become acutely aware of where I stand, of the space I occupy. I hesitate. The tension is there, familiar. The fear of being too much, of taking up too much space, of breaking some unspoken rule. And at the same time, the fear of not being enough.

Still, I open my mouth. The first sound is tentative, caught between restraint and release. Behind me, scattered voices rise and fall, carried by the wind. I wonder if they, too, are caught in the same tension—between excess and absence, between needing to be heard and fearing what their voice might reveal. A breath drawn deep, a voice rising, moving through my body, vibrating in my chest, leaving me weightless for a moment as I expand with the sound into the open landscape. A release—not just of sound, but of something deeper, something I didn't know I was holding.

I scream, not in anger, not in despair, but simply to feel my presence, to mark that I am here. That I exist beyond the roles, beyond expectation. For a moment, the landscape is filled with us. Not as doctors, not as anything defined, just bodies, breath, sound. The ocean does not answer, but it receives.

Then silence again. The sea, the wind, the world unchanged. And yet, something in me is different.

Edvin: In the Nordic languages, to vote is "to voice." A decision is "a voicing." Metaphors are telling. To use my voice is to exert authority as an individual by claiming attention. People can avert their eyes and pretend not to see, but ears cannot be closed. To raise one's voice is to make oneself noticed. With my voice I claim space and attention. I also claim respect. And respect can only be given by others. By using my voice and exerting my authority I put others in a position to accept or reject me, acknowledge or ignore me, admire or laugh at me. My sound is my audible self. So much safer to just be quiet. So easy not to voice those sounds, or utter those words, that others could judge as ugly, jarring, wrong, stupid.

Caroline: Sharp stones, the coldness of the moss, screaming into open space. A transgression of the boundaries of collectives and their norms, a confrontation with the limits of self. That resistance—whether against sound, sensation, or expectation—holds knowledge within it. Coming to voice is not just an intellectual exercise but an embodied one. Voice does not emerge from the endless rehearsal of discourse, from word games. It does not come from the mastery of language alone. It comes from within—from what is felt before it is spoken, from what is known in the body before it is articulated in words. To speak with voice is not to recite but to reveal, not to conform but to make present something real, something lived. To humanize medicine is not only to expand what can be said, but to make space for what must be voiced—not as performance, but as presence. To recognize these limits of language is not to abandon words and stories but to engage with them differently—to acknowledge that knowing is not only about articulation but also about attunement, interpretation, and responsiveness to what cannot be fully said. Medicine, if it is to be humanized, must embrace not only what it can define but also what it must dwell with, listen for, and remain open to.

Edvin: The year-long planning, the attempts to create ways of being together that could disrupt and enlarge conventional means of learning to be a good doctor, stemmed from a dream that somehow, through relating in daring and empowering ways, we would each become better able to see for ourselves, get closer to sources of insight. Wisdom resides in embodied knowledge, in meetings of minds, in disruptive events that jolt us out of complacency. Art can have that effect, of opening doors in your mind, to rooms you have forgotten, or never known existed. The seminar intended to have that effect—to make the familiar strange, force us to wonder, make potentialities tangible, make the future crack open, let in some light.

Caroline: Did we succeed? Here, in this space, hierarchies wavered. Speech was tentative, authority momentarily unsettled. Who speaks. Who listens. Who holds the weight of the conversation. Who gifts and who receives. The seminar, like medicine itself, a site of negotiation, vulnerability, and constraint. A space where care was not just a topic but a practice, unfolding in real time. And like in medicine, the stakes were high—not in life and death, but in the risk of misunderstanding, dismissal, or the failure to hold what needed holding. It was here that detachment was not just discussed but felt—the impulse to retreat, to contain, to keep knowledge at a safe distance. It was here that the weight of care became tangible—not just as an ethical imperative, but as a burden, an obligation, a force that binds and demands. But what happens when medicine, like this seminar, is no longer structured around the avoidance of difficulty, but the practice of staying with it? What is needed?

Edvin: The seminar unfolded through long days of talking, thinking, gonging, shouting, breathing, resting. Gradually, I felt that perceptions, impressions, emotions, and ideas contained in and emerging from the strange events created by this group of living, embodied physicians in search of the right stuff of medicine were woven together. Strands of courage, recognition, respect, relief, deep knowledge, joy, and attachment came together and gave birth to a feeling that was difficult to name. But it felt like strength. Not my individual strength, but the unfamiliar yet recognizable strength of collective effort, judgement, direction. Strength from having honestly struggled with evasive questions about the meaning of life and the goals of medicine, of having experienced and examined shared practices on the bodily, the mental, the relational, and the spiritual levels of being.

It is true that I had been hesitant when Caroline brought up this risky idea about the being sessions. Could we risk hour after hour of improvised contributions from the participants? What about my need for control and predictability? Perhaps it was the realization that I, again, contradicted myself that made me yield. Or perhaps it was Caroline's burning eyes and contagious belief in the idea. Added to that, the trust of courageous colleagues who chose to take part in this undertaking rekindled my old, naïve hope, that somehow, one day, there would come a time when what I know as a person and what I know as a doctor will be allowed to come together.

Caroline: The marbles lying close together in the little glass jar are not just symbols. Small, weighted, tactile, they are disruptive in their very presence. Unlike the rigid structures of hierarchy that often define medicine, the marbles do not assert position, rank, or authority. Each is distinct, yet none is above or below the other. They exist in relation, in movement, exchanged not as possessions but as gestures of recognition, of trust, of shared carrying. They are disruptive, but not destructive. The marbles do not answer. They remain, quiet but insistent, reminding us that care, like knowledge, is always relational. Always at risk. Always in motion.

Edvin and Caroline: We did not answer the question *What Is the Right Stuff of Medicine?* In fact, the knowledge that emerged was not primarily about medicine, but about what it takes to sustain ourselves within it. It was knowledge about what it means— what it takes—to steward medicine—not as something fixed, but as something that must be tended to, questioned, and cared for. To sit with the questions: *How does medicine fail? How do we fail? What does it require of us to be responsible?* Responsibility not just for what we do, but for what we fail to do—for what we overlook, for what we dismiss, for the ways we participate in medicine's harms even as we seek to heal. It was about the courage to stay open, to let thinking be something that is made, together, in real time.

Through presence, exchange, and shared practice, we made tangible certain dimensions of strength required for care. Care—not as passive acts of benevolence, but as a relationship that necessitates negotiation, discernment, and responsibility. We exposed and engaged with what is at stake and what is required to care for medicine, to expand ways of knowing in medicine, to humanize medicine.

Care is not just given; it is wielded. It can heal, but it can also impose, constrain, and control.

Care takes curiosity—an openness to what is not yet understood, with the humility to recognize when curiosity itself becomes intrusive.

Care takes courage—to risk uncertainty and stay with discomfort, but also to know when the courage to act turns into the arrogance of knowing best.

Care takes attunement—to recognize what is unspoken and needed, but also to acknowledge that attunement is never pure, that power shapes whose voices are listened to and whose are ignored.

Care takes receptivity—to receive without absorbing, to listen without rushing to respond, but also to know that to receive is not always to accept—that refusal, too, is a form of care.

Care takes steadiness—to navigate responsibility without disappearing into detachment, but also to resist the steadiness that is rigidity, that rejects what does not fit with your ways of knowing.

Each being session, each gesture of exchange, each moment of silence, each offering of presence was a small enactment of these tensions, symbolized by a little sphere of stone. The act of exchange—a marble from one hand to another—disrupts the usual flows of knowledge and authority in medicine. Here, knowledge was not something extracted, codified, or imposed, but something entrusted.

The being sessions were reminders that care is not just something we do, but something we enact within systems of power. That knowledge is not just something we possess, but something we shape. That care is not neutral, that stewardship is not abstract. That to care is to make decisions about what matters, and for whom.

A tiny glass jar. Thirteen colourful, polished stones, each carrying weight beyond its size. Each one representing a person, a presence, an offering. Each one a remembrance of practice, knowledge, connection, care, strength. Together, they form a token of responsibility—of what has been carried and of what must be held.

References

Bargh, J. A., & Chartrand, T. L. (1999). The unbearable automaticity of being. *American Psychologist, 54*(7), 462.

Fleck, L. (1979). Genesis and development of a scientific fact. In F. Bradley & T. J. Trenn (Eds.), *Theories of social order*. Chicago University Press.

Foucault, M. (1975). *The birth of the clinic: An archaeology of medical perception*. Random House.

Gibran, K. (1923). *The prophet*. Alfred A. Knopf.

Good, B. J. (1994). *Medicine, rationality, and experience: An anthropological perspective*. Cambridge University Press.

Hafferty, F. W. (2016). Socialization, professionalism, and professional identity formation. In R. L. Cruess, S. R. Cruess, & Y. Steinert (Eds.), *Teaching medical professionalism* (2nd ed., pp. 54–67). Cambridge University Press.

Hayles, N. K. (2014). Cognition everywhere: The rise of the cognitive nonconscious and the costs of consciousness. *New Literary History, 45*(2), 199–220.

Kemmis, S. (2012). Phronesis, experience, and the primacy of praxis. In E. A. Kinsella & A. Pitman (Eds.), *Phronesis as professional knowledge: Practical wisdom in the professions* (pp. 147–162). SensePublishers. Imprint. http://dx.doi.org/10.1007/978-94-6091-731-8

Nisbett, R. E., & Wilson, T. D. (1977). Telling more than we can know: Verbal reports on mental processes. *Psychological Review, 84*(3), 231–259. https://doi.org/10.1037/0033-295X.84.3.231

Polanyi, M. (1966). *The tacit dimension*. Doubleday & Co.

Schei, E., Fuks, A., & Boudreau, J. D. (2019, 2019/06/01). Reflection in medical education: Intellectual humility, discovery, and know-how. *Medicine, Health Care and Philosophy, 22*(2), 167–178. https://doi.org/10.1007/s11019-018-9878-2

Wenger, E. (1998). *Communities of practice: Learning, meaning, and identity*. Cambridge University Press.

11

I'll Take It with Me When I Go

Knut Eirik Eliassen

When I woke up this morning and pulled back the curtains, the same feeling washed over me as it did yesterday—this could be home! Despite traveling for more than 12 hours to reach this cabin on the edge of the Atlantic, with Hebridean islets scattered like jewels between us and Greenland. These islets change their hues with the weather, turning green to yellow when the sun pierces through the dense clouds and shifting from brown to grey during rainstorms. Closing my eyes and opening them again, I could easily imagine being by the Sognefjord in Norway.

I blink away a headache. The air is crisp. The still fjord mirrors the morning sun. I briefly consider a wake-up swim.

It's easy to imagine how Vikings and their descendants pulled their boats ashore here and that seeds stuck under their boots found soil to sprout in, making the vegetation above the rocks along the shoreline similar to the trees and bushes at home. The ocean outside my window was once the highway for travel and trade between Norway and Scotland. I picture sturdy women onboard—so strong that the Scottish clansmen who married them let them keep their maiden names, as evidenced by the old tombs in the churchyards of Edinburgh.

I hear quiet activity in the kitchen below and glance at my watch. Through the window I glimpse a badger sneaking home to his den, the bushes rustling a little. I forget my dreams, but the feeling remains—a calmness this morning. The silent sound of night fades as the early birds greet the light.

DOI: 10.1201/9781003593294-11

Jack the cook is already up. The homely scent of yeast fills my nostrils. The burnt aroma of ground coffee beans motivates me to get up. The care he shows for us allows us to focus on thinking, being, and exploring our tasks and questions both alone and together. I slink down the stairs, nod a quiet "good morning," and raise my coffee mug in greeting. I glimpse one of the other participants wrapped in a woollen blanket in a lounge chair on the terrace—getting her coffee and calmly contemplating her own being before the rest are up.

I sneak back to my room, open my window, and climb under my sheets. Morning coffee with a view and in silent solitude. Not too many mornings are like these, an hour of being, one that isn't in my calendar.

Had it been completely up to me—and maybe it is—every morning would have room for contemplation. About yesterday and tomorrow. Then about today. Could I just *be*, for once?

As my brain adapts to the morning light and absorbs the caffeine, I realize why my thoughts are wandering. Today is my "being session" day. We have all been asked, *What keeps you going? What increases your carrying capacity?* One of those things, for me, is to catch a song when I hear it. Some songs I learn by heart, to collect them in my gem box, and keep them with me.

An hour later, I am dressed, full from freshly baked bread and fried eggs, and it's my turn. I'm not nervous, although I had expected to be. I feel completely calm.

Preparing for a larger talk, lecture, or teaching, I am always nervous, and I cherish the moment in my preparations when I am not yet done but can say to myself that had it been now—I would have managed. From that moment on, my nerves sharpen my concentration, and I often feel a quiet calmness and presence.

The clock strikes nine. I open the double sliding doors to the terrace and ask all my co-participants to turn towards the sea. The fresh morning air fills the room. A seagull cries in the distance, and we hear the waves gently striking the shore, making the smallest pebbles on the beach whirl around. I now look at the backs of 13 morning-fresh heads. Instead of having them stare at me and making me uneasy, they rest their eyes on the scenery. *"Good morning, welcome to my being session. I have come to the conclusion that what helps me is using my brain in a different way."*

Then I sing.

147

12

Alienation, Resonance, and the Formation of Physicians

Edvin Schei

Physician philosopher Eric Cassell wrote in 2012: "I believe that clinicians, no matter how much they want to be patient centered or focus on healing, do not really know how to do it" (Cassell, 2012). In this chapter, I will examine Cassell's claim and how it relates to medical education, in particular to the types of professional knowledge and the tacit understanding of doctoring that medical learners develop.

Eric Cassell was an enthusiastic primary care clinician. He worked for more than 40 years as an internist in New York City, meeting sick people from all layers of society. Early on, he realized that although as a physician he knew a lot about disease, that knowledge did not allow him to truly help his sickest and most desperate patients, such as a young mother dying of breast cancer, to whom the medicine of the 1960s had little to offer. Then, as now, many patients appeared "difficult" to their physicians because they suffered, not just from somatic dysfunction but from losses and threats on three other dimensions of life—their relationships to the world around them, their personal goals and purposes, and their experience of overarching existential meaning (Cassell, 2004).

Cassell noticed that if he talked to his patients with real curiosity and got to know them as persons, not just as diseased bodies, he would often be able to provide help. Indeed, his interest in the patients' lives and troubles seemed often to be helpful in itself. Inspired by this understanding, he published

DOI: 10.1201/9781003593294-12

books on clinical communication (Cassell, 1985), learned how to perform hypnosis and applied it as part of cancer treatment, and studied philosophy to learn more than medical school had taught him about people, logic, and meaning. Informed by these perspectives, Cassell published a ground-breaking article in the *New England Journal of Medicine* in 1982, entitled "The Nature of Suffering and the Goals of Medicine." It has been cited more than 5000 times in scientific publications and marked the beginning of medicine's research interest in suffering. Cassell has been recognized as one of the founders of palliative medicine. He died in 2021.

So, what led Cassell to claim that clinicians "do not really know" how to be patient-centred or focus on healing? I will argue that Cassell's observation is largely correct and that it points to knowledge gaps and misunderstandings within mainstream medicine and medical education which have wide-ranging consequences for patients, physicians, and society (Stewart et al., 2024).

I feel in a good position to interpret Eric Cassell's philosophy of medicine. For nearly 20 years, he was a mentor and close friend. I spent weeks in his house, deep in a walnut forest in Pennsylvania, surrounded by books, deer, and wild turkeys. In front of the fireplace, we would talk about life, medicine, our patients, our own attempts to understand. Eric was deeply fascinated by medicine. "I love disease," he would say. "I've come to learn, however, that the central phenomenon in medicine is not disease. It's the person. But physicians don't learn about persons. Diagnosis is the law of gravity in medicine. That's why we so often fail to help those who suffer."

Medical Success, Medical Trouble

We live in times of great medical achievements; for over a century, medicine has offered biological exploration and technological innovation. As a result, every day, lives worth saving are being saved and horrible human suffering is relieved or prevented.

Yet ours are also times of dissatisfaction and disappointment with health-care; of underfunded and understaffed medical institutions, unfair distribution of health services, and greedy parasitism on people's vulnerabilities by "health" business and technology that waste resources and cause harm through medical overdiagnosis. And we are in the midst of an epidemic of burnt-out doctors and medical students across the world (Dyrbye & Shanafelt, 2016).

Medicine is no island in itself; its problems are deeply enmeshed within the societal and historical dynamics of the age we live in, often called "late modernity" (see Chapter 3). In secularized societies, medicine is the guide that people trust in questions of health, sickness, and suffering. The medical schools not only define what a "real doctor" needs to know, they indirectly provide the public with theories and recipes for how certain universal problems—those concerning bodily and existential vulnerability in life and death—should be framed and addressed. As young persons enter university and learn to become doctors, they bring with them lay assumptions about what doctors know and do. Those assumptions are not fundamentally challenged at the universities; rather, they are reinforced as students embody "the clinical gaze" (Foucault, 1975). Over generations, the stereotypically medical way of viewing and stewarding life has become a dominant impulse in societies at large, shaping expectations and actions that build health—or fail in the attempt to do so.

With the sudden advent of revolutionizing technologies such as the internet, the smartphone, and artificial intelligence, the world has accelerated into a frenzied pace of communication and information. This has also had a profound effect on the speed with which social values and possibilities change. Problems in healthcare, including physicians' alienation and burnout, are part of these upheavals.

Medicine and medical education cannot stem the tide of societal transformation. But it is medicine's task to examine and understand how suffering emerges in our times and to train helpers who can cure, care, comfort, and heal. What do doctors need to learn, think, feel and be able to do, to, in Cassell's words "be patient centered or focus on healing?"

Knowledge Treating Disease?

Over the course of my lifetime in medicine, as student, clinician, educator, researcher, author, patient, and relative, I have oscillated between admiration and loathing of the profession and its cultural universe. I have felt guilty for criticizing a highly lauded endeavour and for offending courageous colleagues who hold out in the trenches of clinical care. I have also been humbled by realizing that I often struggle to live up to the high ideals of a clinician that Eric Cassell honoured and that I share.

Troubled by such contradictions, and inspired by thousands of encounters with patients and students, I have searched for broader knowledge and better doctoring skills, hoping to develop a more helpful understanding of sickness, suffering, and medical work. I wanted more than the heroic clichés of doctoring-as-problem-fixing that filled my toolbox when I was a beginner, the same commonplaces that were taught to my mentor Eric Cassell, and to all doctors since the beginning of the twentieth century, when natural science transformed medicine.

The perception of doctors as heroic body-fixers may have been there since the dawn of time, expressing humanity's hopes and wishful thinking when faced with sickness and death. However, with medicine's astounding technical developments over the last century, expectations of miraculous cures and remedies have intensified. At the core of medicine's technical successes lies the mechanical assumption, going back at least to Descartes in the sixteenth century, that we can help sick people with similar principles that we use to repair faulty machines: We find out why it doesn't work and try to fix the broken part. Medical students are taught that a living organism can be understood through knowing its parts, that sick persons are healed by curing their diseases, and that mind and body are distinct realms. Thus, each new generation of physicians is trained to approach the job as—well-behaved and compassionate—mechanics of broken bodies.

The mechanical understanding of the body, of health and sickness, and of what doctors should be able to do is the taken-for-granted worldview of Western healthcare. Its assumptions are what in philosophical parlance can be called "the tacit ontology and epistemology of modern medicine" (Pellegrino & Thomasma, 1981). It can even be summarized in a formula: "Medicine is knowledge treating disease."

This formula captures how each clinician is reduced to an exchangeable carrier of knowledge and each patient to a vehicle of disease. This instrumental approach is not wrong; it saves lives when a heart stops or a wound bleeds profusely. But it is greatly insufficient and dangerous when misapplied. "An exquisite understanding of disease cannot explain why the patient is sick any more than the formula H_2O can tell you why water is wet," writes Cassell (Cassell, 2012, p. 55). The successes of technical medicine have even marginalized other kinds of medical knowledge. Attempts to gain insight into feelings, values, relationships, and purpose in life—the pillars of the patient's existence—can seem trivial or irrelevant to the doctor who thinks their job is to make diagnoses and treat disease (Cassell, 2004).

Actually, it *is* a doctor's job to make diagnoses and treat disease. Without diagnostic knowledge, a clinician is useless. *But* it is far from enough: For each heart that stops, cancer that is cured, or life that is saved, there are 10,000 consultations where the physician meets patients who need help with symptoms and dysfunctions that never go away. Patients with sadness, aches, and pains; with shortness of breath, fatigue, and sleeping problems; with worries about the gruelling job, the violent spouse, or the demented parents; with addiction, personality disorders, side effects of migraine medication, vaccines, or cancer treatment. Every day, doctors meet patients who demand tests, imaging, sick leaves, and pills that are not good for them. And then there are the patients who are lonely, poor, and miserable, whose sources of joy and resilience have dried out—who seek doctors because their bodies seem to betray them and who do not know that body, mind, and relations shape each other, in health and sickness (see Chapter 6). Normal people, like my recent patient Anne.

Disease Only Comes in the Form of Sick People

Anne, a vibrant 20 year old, strides into the emergency room with quick, purposeful steps. She meets my gaze and offers a firm handshake. Her well-groomed appearance and confident demeanour suggest efficiency and self-assurance. With a resigned sigh she lets me know that she has yet another urinary tract infection. I glance at her notes and see that it has only been a few weeks since her last visit for the same issue. I ask if she has had frequent antibiotic treatments. She lifts her eyes, ponders for a moment, and then, with a flat voice, says "Yes, maybe 25 times in the last year, for cystitis and throat infections."

I am startled by this information. What is it that makes Anne so susceptible to infections? Does she have a bladder cancer or immune failure? For a healthy-looking 20 year old, a purely biological explanation is unlikely. I invite Anne to tell me a little about her life and who she is. A lengthy conversation and shedding of tears ensue. Anne was diagnosed with depression at 12. She suffers from irritable bowel syndrome with frequent bouts of constipation and abdominal pain. Her childhood was tumultuous, her mother an alcoholic. The family fell apart when Anne was 11, forcing her into a parental role for her parents and two younger sisters. She lets me understand that she has been sexually abused. Anne is very good at hiding her loneliness and despair. She had mentioned to her GP that she might need to see a psychologist, but the GP, looking tired and dejected, had suggested, "Let's take one thing at a time and try to fix the bodily issues first, OK?"

Hearing this story, one hardly needs a medical degree to intuit that Anne's bodily problems may be related to her life situation, to her personality, her values, her suffering, the harm to her immune system caused by long-standing fear, shame, defensiveness, and the toxic levels of stress hormones that such emotions entail.

But gaining the young woman's trust, seeking out the hidden stories, piecing together evidence of recurring infections with theory about emotion, brain function, and immunity so that a narrative can be constructed of which the patient herself was completely unaware yet becomes willing to acknowledge and can use for therapeutic change—that takes professional competence.

Stories like Anne's are written in invisible ink and remain illegible to doctors who are guided by the disease model of medicine and have been trained to solve problems by zooming in on the manifest symptoms, the infections, the choice of treatments, the unlikely but not impossible existence of some hidden biological pathology. While trying to fix Anne's health problems by targeting her diseases one by one, doctors run the risk of harming Anne's prospects for life by making her story and its meaning irrelevant, invisible, and incomprehensible.

And doctors who try yet fail to help their patients suffer too.

Physicians Are Also People

In today's landscapes of healthcare, more than 50% of young hospital physicians (West et al., 2018) and about a third of family doctors (Hiefner et al., 2022) show signs of burnout. What does that mean? It means that thousands and thousands of conscientious, idealistic, and hard-working individuals go to their daily work as helpers of people in a state of emotional depletion, not really able to feel engagement or compassion, perceiving patients as cases and diagnostic challenges without being touched by them as suffering individuals. Physicians with burnout are weighed down by their own suffering. They are constantly tired, their energy levels are low, they have a diminished sense of personal achievement and competence, they have doubts about the quality and impact of their work and qualms about being personally inadequate (see Chapters 2 and 15). At its most severe, burnout impairs cognitive function and decision making and increases the risk of physician errors, of substance abuse and suicide. What pushes so many idealistic young people into that morass?

Explanations for the plague of despair and mental pain among clinicians have been found in the harsh work environments of hospitals, in constant job stress, in physician's perfectionism and moral distress, and in the gradual emotional corrosion caused by compassion fatigue, helplessness and disgust in close encounters with sick, decaying, and suffering persons who cannot be fixed. But if these are the flames that consume doctors' joy and vitality, what causes the heat underneath; what is the fuel?

The main suspect is loss of meaning—alienation (Engen, 2025). Psychiatrist Viktor Frankl survived Auschwitz and posited man's experience of meaning (Frankl, 1946) as the main source of mental health, a view shared by philosopher Friedrich Nietzsche who once famously claimed that "He who has a *why* to live for can bear almost any how." How does "meaning" manifest in the tough everyday life of healthcare work? People will put up with the unavoidable wear and tear of human misery, frustrating workplaces, and imperfect learning environments as long as they have a sense of purpose, a sense of belonging, and a secure knowledge that their personal efforts matter and are appreciated (Deci & Ryan, 2008; Flett, 2022).

Too often, however, physicians are left without the rewards of being appreciated and of feeling that they matter because they work in a system where medicine is taught, assessed, and practised not as a meaning-making endeavour between persons, that which Cassell calls "healing," but as "knowledge treating disease"—bare industrial biomedicine. Within this logic it does not matter WHO the physician is, as long as the accurate diagnosis leads to the correct algorithm for treatment. For the idealistic young doctor who wants to make a difference in people's lives, who wants to matter as a trusted helper, a valued colleague, and a likable human being, it is disorienting to find that little more is expected of them than to be a useful cogwheel in a factory of diagnostic processes and predetermined routines. Expectations of affecting and being affected, of resonance with patients and their healing processes, are subtly unmet, and meaning erodes (Schei, 2006). "When their efforts to act responsibly are frustrated, when they find themselves unable to use their faculties, humans suffer," wrote Paulo Freire (Freire, 1970/2017, p. 51).

As a junior resident on call I received a very sick toddler with signs of infection. I looked up the recommended diagnostic tests, interpreted the results as indicating bacterial meningitis, looked up the correct treatment regimen, and ordered the nurses to carry it out. The child's life was saved. But I was left with a dull feeling of guilt. Not for doing anything wrong, but for my complete lack of pride and joy, even a lack of compassion with the parents. It felt as if I had done nothing more than exercise my ability to read an algorithm and unleash the knowledge it contained. My personal contribution, as the thinking, creative, compassionate individual I wanted to be, seemed trivial. I realized that the dramatic events were not about me. But I couldn't help it, I wanted to matter more, I felt empty.

After a year of hospital doctoring, trying to incarnate "knowledge treating disease," I considered quitting medicine entirely. I was alienated, probably, though I had no name for my reaction at the time. It took years to redis-cover the joy and enthusiasm of being a doctor, years of listening to stories, of reading outside of medicine, seeking out knowledge about the living body and the human condition, fumblingly trying out the healing powers of the physician role, and reflecting with wiser people—Eric Cassell one of them—about life and death, about what can be meaningfully changed and what is better left untouched by medicine. This voyage eventually restored my sense of purpose as a physician and changed my approach to clinical work. As I learned more, I felt less confined to focus always on diagnostics and categorization of patients and their problems, more able to complement the disease-centred approach with a caring exploration of sick persons' experiences, resources, and purposes in life. I found myself more often able to offer help by facilitating other's healing processes, such as change, eman-cipation, or reconciliation with loss and limits (Schei, 2006). The realiza-tion that there are powerful ways of doing medicine which medical school had not taught me kindled my interest in medical education, in what goes on in medical schools. It seemed clear that the cradle where each new gen-eration learns how to feel, think, and act like a physician is the university.

Education as Enlightenment or Brainwashing

Education in the professions is often understood as mere qualification, a gruelling but rather mechanical, year-long accumulation of capability in brains and hands of learners who remain essentially the same persons. But that is not what happens. Education involves a deep transformation of learn-ers' perceived worlds, of their values, their approach to problem solving, and their emotional reactions to breaches of unpronounced professional norms (Valestrand, 2024). The change process that gradually transforms newcomers into old-timers is called socialization; it is effected through non-conscious adoption of language and opinions displayed by important others such as peers and professors, and it manifests as subtle changes in students' automated habits of perception, language, emotion, and action, which eventually lead each individual to think, feel, and act in ways that share traits and are somehow "typical" of physicians (Bargh & Chartrand, 1999; Hafferty, 2016). Yet, for education to really succeed, we want more than qualification and socialization; we want autonomous judgement and agency (Biesta & van Braak, 2023; Schei et al., 2019). This is the realm of "subjectification," of becoming a subject in one's own life, with the freedom "to say yes or to say no, to stay or to walk away, to go with the flow or to resist," as educational philosopher Gert Biesta writes (Biesta, 2020, p. 93). Subjectification "is about how I exist as the subject of my own life, not as the object of what other people want from me" (Biesta, 2020, p. 93).

In medical education, subjectification does not figure among the learning goals. In 2018, I and a group of colleagues published an interview study (Schei et al., 2018) investigating the process of professional identity formation after one year at Bergen medical school. In group interviews, the young students described the ideal physician as a caring person with unusual moral strength, who can "do things that are not expected of ordinary people, in a way." About their learning needs, one student said: "I feel that to learn how to be humane is almost as important as learning about disease." When asked how the university helped them become this kind of physician, their replies displayed two contradictory perspectives, one critical and the other apologetic. "There is a lot of human contact in being a physician, and it surprises me that there's so much theory and so little human contact. It's as if we are being educated to see the human being as a machine, a biological machine." Reflecting on the school's influence on their independence, a student said, "When you enter medical school it's maybe a little frightening, and. . . . You'll accept anything, you don't dare to object against them. It's like you go through a factory, and you end up a product of that factory." Such criticism was balanced, however, often by the same students, by statements displaying trust in the wisdom of the system: "You learn it later, you find out later what is important"; belief that knowledge is protective: "I think it's fine to know some anatomy before you sort of have to talk to patients"; and the maturing effects of figuring things out for oneself: "You have to grow up at some stage."

The article concludes that the students are at risk of being brainwashed into conformity with a professional world where knowledge is what can be memorized and assessed and where critical thinking, self-awareness, and emotions are suppressed (Shapiro, 2011). Sadly paradoxical, education seems to foster "impoverished critical thinking, naïve objectivism and deficient understanding both of biomedical science and of how clinicians use knowledge, as well as alienation and suppression of emotion, producing burnout and cynicism" (Schei et al., 2018). The results are congruent with the Carnegie Foundation's report on American medical education, stating that traditional teaching models invite "learning strategies such as rote memorization that are inimical to scientific reasoning and inquiry" (Cooke et al., 2010). Or as philosopher and mathematician Bertrand Russel quipped—"Men are born ignorant, not stupid. They are made stupid by education."

Curricular reforms at my university, Bergen medical school, have in later years tried to mitigate the weaknesses of the medical study program. But as new pedagogical goals are introduced, the teaching staff remains the same—researchers and academic clinicians steeped in the traditional conception of disease-centred medicine, using old-style methods of knowledge transmission and high-stakes assessment. In 2024, fifth-year student Emilie Aase did a survey of 600 Bergen students, finding that more than 40% had symptoms of burnout or depression. In a separate project using autoethnography to explore the medical school experience, Eldrid Nilsen, a fourth-year student with extensive experience as an elected representative of the student community, writes (2024, personal communication):

Dear medical school. You want me to become like you. A shadow of myself. Afraid to stand up for what I believe is right. Afraid to say something wrong. Always worried that time is running out. Thinking that I must become infallible. Hide my own humanity. And you have succeeded with far too many. Overworked. Gray-faced. Tired. Joyless. Muffled. Vulnerable, imperfect, fantastically skilled. They keep you going. You don't understand what it costs them. But I see it. It costs too much.
I've lived in the belief that as long as I speak up about what doesn't work, those responsible will take care of it. I've been speaking to deaf ears for years. And it does something to me.

Good Life, Resonance, and the Healing Encounter

Some academics claim that "what is a good life" is not a scientific question, since any answer is bound to be value-laden and relative, saturated with history and culture. But recent trends in the social sciences dispute this nihilist view, claiming that professionals need a language for talking about what constitutes a good life in order to identify widespread social phenomena that undermine health and well-being.

The title of this chapter alludes to the concept of "resonance." The salience of resonance in current critical theory can be attributed to German sociologist Hartmut Rosa. He understands resonance to be life-sustaining and growth-inspiring, the counterforce to slow alienation (Rosa, 2018). Rosa argues that alienation from many causes is at the root of burnout and depression in modern society. Alienation can be defined as the erosion of meaning in people's daily lives. An alienating relationship—be it to humans, work, school or other aspects of one's life-world—is one that lacks "a true, vibrant exchange and connection: between a silent and grey world and a 'dry' subject there is no life, both appear to be either frozen or genuinely chaotic and mutually aversive" (Rosa, 2018). Resonance exists when I feel "touched, moved, or addressed by the people, places, objects" that I encounter. Resonance is the realization that we actually affect others "and that they truly listen and connect to us and answer in return" (Rosa, 2018). Resonance is not just harmony or a confirming echo of my own voice. It is to be affected by that which is beyond my control and speaks in its own voice or key, be it in encounters with nature, beauty, work, or persons. Being touched by and responding to this alien voice entails a moment of self-transcendence, of stepping into unknowns. Thus, resonance is life changing. And it cannot be controlled or predicted. There is never a guarantee that an encounter will have resonance; I can only create the best conditions for it to happen.

Can failure to foster "resonance" be a key to understanding Eric Cassell's claim that "clinicians, no matter how much they want to be patient-centred or focus on healing, do not really know how to do it"? I think so. Essential to patient-centred practice, and at the core of any act of healing, is the resonance that can emerge in an encounter between two human subjects with different worlds, needs, and roles, joined in an effort to alleviate suffering (Stewart et al., 2024). From that resonance come trust, compassion, understanding, hope, motivation, and reconciliation. The encounters within clinical medicine will be more or less transient, more or less instrumental, more or less reciprocal, all depending on the context, the nature of the health problem, and who those two persons are. But good medicine is never just "a problem" that needs "a fix." There will always be a human being at each end of a healing encounter, and both will be affected by it, both will be jolted, changed, or energized by the transcendent effects of the resonance that occurs. "The individual never has anything to do with another human being without holding something of that person's life in their hands," wrote Danish philosopher Knud Løgstrup (Løgstrup, 1997). In the age of AI, much will change that can make the opposite seem more and more true. But the machines, be they robots or clinicians who are alienated or brainwashed, do not know how to heal.

To educate competent biomedical doctors who are able to foster resonance with their patients, medical education must allow learners to bring the wisdom of their subjective life experience into the professional realm. "Health workers who deeply understand what it is for themselves to be healthy are more likely to empathize with the health experiences of others," writes medical philosopher Stan van Hooft (van Hooft, 1997). He points out that a clinician can only grasp the meaning of someone else's loss of health if she is aware of how she experiences her own health and what it is that makes health "important and valuable." It is in the shared experience of lifelong vulnerable subjectivity that sufferer and healer can resonate across all cultural and hierarchical differences and barriers. And this resonance between doctor and patient can replenish meaning lost to sickness and isolation and energize change, adaptation, and reconciliation—which are facets of healing.

A Nod, a Smile, a Name

I end this chapter with a sunny story about creating conditions for resonance to happen.

It started in 2019 with a research study where we interviewed groups of senior medical students about experiences of shame. They all had examples of being shamed during clinical placements. The recurring theme was not harassment and bullying, but a chilly learning environment where too many physicians did not seem to welcome or care about students, who often felt "like dirt under someone's shoe," as a student said (Whelan et al., 2021).

Our informants recalled doctors who would not make eye contact when greeting them and supervisors who told students they had no tasks for them to take part in while having their backs turned towards them. A student said: *"I think it's about body language. . . . If someone says 'Leonard, you should be with this doctor today' and* [the doctor] *just walks away, it's very hard. You need to look someone in the eyes to say hello to them"* (Valestrand et al., 2024).

Students were often not addressed as a person, but with a generic "student." *"Can the student leave the room!"* The effect on students' agency and learning was strongly negative: *"My professionalism and my ability to be a good med student and a good doctor are connected to confidence. This whole process gets thrown off if someone comes in and shakes that little confidence that you have. It's much harder to launch yourself into something new if you don't know if anyone is there to catch you."*

In 2021, we started a pilot project, PROFMED, to see if we could improve the clinical learning environment by preparing medical students for their practice periods and somehow change negative attitudes and improve supervisory skills among hospital doctors. We knew it was a complex project with many pitfalls and invited researchers from six universities in Norway, Canada, the UK, and Sweden. Ambitions were high. But as we got down to the realities on the ground, we soon learned that it wouldn't be easy. Like most hospitals, the one we selected for our intervention was understaffed, and clinicians were overworked and not unfamiliar with burnout. The clinicians expressed interest in the project but made it clear that they could not contribute by dedicating time. Our dreams of carefully educating the physicians to become skilled clinical supervisors rapidly crumbled.

What we also learned was that the students' main contacts were not senior clinicians, but the young residents who spent time in the emergency rooms and on the wards. Among these, we were eventually able to recruit a handful of volunteers on the condition that involvement in the project would not cost them any additional work, time, or stress. So, what could we achieve while keeping that promise?

One thing that does not demand work, time, or stress is to *relate*. The shame study had unveiled the destructive impact of physician supervisors' non-relating. Would it be possible to change that? Doctors are well-intentioned people but seemed to lack awareness of the power of their role. We had learned from sociolinguistic and anthropological theory why greetings were so powerful (Laver, 1975). They convey information about the speakers' identities, attitudes, and relative rank. The more powerful participant, such as a physician supervisor, may greet first to give the other "safe conduct to enter his territory without making him suffer a counter display of hostility" (Laver, 1975). Using the other's name triggers brain activity that facilitates attachment (Carmody & Lewis, 2006).

Ritual behaviour and small talk that signal friendliness are called "phatic communication" (Laver, 1975). Phatic functions of language make it possible for strangers to relate without fear. Phatic behaviours are tools "for the detailed management of interpersonal relationships during the psychologically crucial margins of interaction" (Laver, 1975). Phatic communication, then, is a gateway to resonance. Could we make it work in the hectic hospital environment where inexperienced students meet busy clinicians, sick people, relatives, and staff of many kinds?

Our group of young volunteer physicians had no trouble recognizing their own experiences in the student quotes from the shame study. During a day of training, we reflected together on how things could be changed. Instead of distributing ten students randomly in a department with 50 unprepared physicians, we created "families" by pairing two volunteer supervisors and connecting these with two or three named students. Next, we convinced these diligent physicians that they need not "teach" their students or fill their knowledge gaps; students have other sources for that: "Relax, you are not their teachers, mothers or secretaries." Inviting the students into the doctors' daily run of the mill and giving them tasks and responsibility would be enough, we promised, with research evidence to back the claim (Dornan et al., 2019).

The rest is history. Four years later the project is over, but the PROFMED approach to student supervision continues in the hospital. None of the residents who eventually were enrolled in the program have withdrawn. They report that pedagogic attitudes towards students have radically improved in the department at large. The benefits reaped by supervisors are that students quickly become able to relieve their workload, that they experience pride when they see students become enthusiastic and confident, and that the relation with students makes their job feel fun and meaningful. "It's strange. When we had students before PROFMED, it was just a blur of faces, I don't remember any of them. Now, I remember them as individuals long after they have left."

We have of course monitored the students' experiences closely. We have learned that the "families" and the pairing of students is important initially, then quickly becomes a largely unnoticed backdrop in a safe atmosphere where students find the courage to connect with doctors and nurses, engage in patient work, and share the table with senior physicians during lunch time, something previously unthinkable. The shame narratives have vanished from our interview data. Instead, we hear stories of confidence, resilience, and resonance, as illustrated by this quote from a group interview:

> The last four weeks I have felt useful. I have felt that I can come into the ER and say "Hi, I'm gonna take a patient" and they exclaim "that's great!" So, it's that human response, they actually are happy to see you. That's been really nice. We have talked about it today and yesterday, that we are getting more. . . . . That some of them thank us for the work we do. I had not expected that, but it makes me very happy. So, you feel that you have some kind of value in yourself, you're not just trailing behind someone.

The main significance of the PROFMED experiment is not that it made clinical learning more efficient—which it did. Its importance lies in showing that the humanistic concerns discussed in this chapter have practical on-the-ground manifestations, consequences, and remedies. It points to simple, humane ways of countering alienation, finding resonance, and offering care to persons whose lives will be spent caring for others.

Get Closer

To Eric Cassell, the sociological concept of resonance was unknown, but the phenomenon it captures was central to his teaching about how to be a good doctor for suffering persons. I interviewed Eric in 2018 about medicine and the alleviation of suffering. There he said:

> *The suffering patient is alone. Nobody understands them, so they stop trying to tell. The first step towards treating suffering is to get closer and try to become one with that patient. You're there, you're not driven away by their symptoms, you're able to talk to them, you're able to touch them, to examine them, they're not alone. Loneliness is always present in suffering, and you have, knowingly or not, addressed their loneliness.*

(Schei, 2018)

As a patient-centred physician, a healer, I must "get closer." Close enough, attentive enough, self-aware enough, listening enough, for resonance to arise. That resonance connects the sufferer with a less alien world and connects the physician with a sense of purpose and agency.

References

Bargh, J. A., & Chartrand, T. L. (1999). The unbearable automaticity of being. *American Psychologist, 54*(7), 462.

Biesta, G. J. (2020). Risking ourselves in education: Qualification, socialization, and subjectification revisited. *Educational Theory, 70*(1), 89–104. https://doi.org/10.1111/edth.12411

Biesta, G. J., & van Braak, M. (2023). Beyond the medical model: Thinking differently about medical education and medical education research. In *Helping a field see itself* (pp. 9–16). CRC Press.

Carmody, D. P., & Lewis, M. (2006). Brain activation when hearing one's own and others' names. *Brain Research, 1116*(1), 153–158.

Cassell, E. J. (1985). *Talking with patients.* MIT Press.

Cassell, E. J. (2004). *The nature of suffering and the goals of medicine* (2nd ed.). Oxford University Press.

Cassell, E. J. (2012). *The nature of healing: The modern practice of medicine*. Oxford University Press.

Cooke, M., Irby, D. M., O'Brien, B. C., & Carnegie Foundation for the Advancement of Teaching. (2010). *Educating physicians: A call for reform of medical school and residency* (1st ed.). Jossey-Bass.

Deci, E. L., & Ryan, R. M. (2008). Self-determination theory: A macrotheory of human motivation, development, and health. *Canadian Psychology/Psychologie canadienne, 49*(3), 182–185. https://doi.org/10.1037/a0012801

Dornan, T., Conn, R., Monaghan, H., Kearney, G., Gillespie, H., & Bennett, D. (2019). Experience based learning (ExBL): Clinical teaching for the twenty-first century. *Medical Teacher, 41*(10), 1098–1105. https://doi.org/10.1080/0142159X.2019.1630730

Dyrbye, L., & Shanafelt, T. (2016). A narrative review on burnout experienced by medical students and residents. *Medical Education, 50*(1), 132–149. https://doi.org/10.1111/medu.12927

Engen, C. (2025). "Doctors must live": A care ethics inquiry into physicians' late modern suffering. *Medicine, Health Care and Philosophy*, 1–16.

Flett, G. L. (2022). An introduction, review, and conceptual analysis of mattering as an essential construct and an essential way of life. *Journal of Psychoeducational Assessment, 40*(1), 3–36.

Foucault, M. (1975). *The birth of the clinic: An archaeology of medical perception*. Random House.

Frankl, V. E. (1946). *Man's search for meaning*. Arneberg Forlag.

Freire, P. (2017). *Pedagogy of the oppressed*. Penguin. (Original work published 1970)

Hafferty, F. W. (2016). Socialization, professionalism, and professional identity formation. In R. L. Cruess, S. R. Cruess, & Y. Steinert (Eds.), *Teaching medical professionalism* (2nd ed., pp. 54–67). Cambridge University Press.

Hiefner, A. R., Constable, P., Ross, K., Sepdham, D., & Ventimiglia, J. B. (2022). Protecting family physicians from burnout: Meaningful patient-physician relationships are "more than just medicine". *The Journal of the American Board of Family Medicine, 35*(4), 716–723. https://doi.org/10.3122/jabfm.2022.04.210441

Laver, J. (1975). Communicative functions of phatic communion. *Organization of Behavior in Face-to-Face Interaction, 215*, 238.

Løgstrup, K. E. (1997). *The ethical demand*. University of Notre Dame Press.

Pellegrino, E. D., & Thomasma, D. C. (1981). *A philosophical basis of medical practice: Toward a philosophy and ethic of the healing professions*. Oxford University Press.

Rosa, H. (2018). The idea of resonance as a sociological concept. *Global Dialogue, 8*(2), 41–44.

Schei, E. (2006). Doctoring as leadership: The power to heal. *Perspectives in Biology and Medicine, 49*(3), 393–406. https://w2.uib.no/filearchive/leadership-schei.pdf

Schei, E. (2018). *Suffering and the modern practice of medicine: A conversation with Eric Cassell*. Omsorg.

Schei, E., Fuks, A., & Boudreau, J. D. (2019). Reflection in medical education: Intellectual humility, discovery, and know-how. *Medicine, Health Care and Philosophy, 22*(2), 167–178. https://doi.org/10.1007/s11019-018-9878-2

Schei, E., Johnsrud, R. E., Mildestvedt, T., Pedersen, R., & Hjörleifsson, S. (2018). Trustingly bewildered: How first-year medical students make sense of their learning experience in a traditional, preclinical curriculum. *Medical Education Online, 23*(1), 1500344. https://doi.org/10.1080/10872981.2018.1500344

Shapiro, J. (2011). Perspective: Does medical education promote professional alexithymia? A call for attending to the emotions of patients and self in medical training. *Academic Medicine, 86*(3), 326–332. https://doi.org/10.1097/ACM.0b013e3182088833

Stewart, M., Brown, J. B., Weston, W. W., Freeman, T., Ryan, B. L., McWilliam, C. L., & McWhinney, I. R. (2024). *Patient-centered medicine: Transforming the clinical method.* CRC Press.

Valestrand, E. A. (2024). *Liminality and transformation: Narrative studies of medical students' and educators' identity processes.* University of Bergen. https://bora.uib.no/bora-xmlui/handle/11250/3147739

Valestrand, E. A., Whelan, B., Eliassen, K. E. R., & Schei, E. (2024). Alienation in the teaching hospital: How physician non-greeting behaviour impacts medical students' learning and professional identity formation. *Perspectives on Medical Education, 13*(1), 239.

van Hooft, S. (1997). Health and subjectivity. *Health, 1*(1), 23–36.

West, C. P., Dyrbye, L. N., & Shanafelt, T. D. (2018). Physician burnout: Contributors, consequences and solutions. *Journal of Internal Medicine, 283*(6), 516–529. https://doi.org/10.1111/joim.12752

Whelan, B., Hjörleifsson, S., & Schei, E. (2021). Shame in medical clerkship: "You just feel like dirt under someone's feet". *Perspectives in Medical Education, 10*(5), 265–271.

Second Thoughts— Reflections on Early Medical Career Experiences

Karl Erik Müller and Caroline Engen

The air is cool, the evening sky streaked with peach and gold. Caroline and Karl Erik slip outside walking towards the sea, leaving the hum of the voices, laughter, and clatter of dishes after dinner. It has been a long day with intense engagement, laughter, some tears, frustration, and—tension.

Outside, under the open sky, the gentle breeze and calming sound of the waves from the sea—this quietness offers something else. A shift and a pause.

Caroline has observed Karl Erik's quietness and puzzlement during some of the discussions during the past days. As they both move farther from the house, the air is filled with a sharp, clean scent of salt and wet rocks. Behind them, the two houses with their tall windows facing the sea catch the last rays of sun, sending flashes of light across the landscape.

Balancing on loose stones, Caroline breaks the silence as she moves towards Karl Erik.

> – I still can't believe how quiet it feels out here. The landscape, the open ocean, the silence. It's a stark contrast to . . . well, everything back home.

DOI: 10.1201/9781003593294-13

Karl Erik walks farther, looking out to the horizon, letting the evening breeze caress his skin.

– Hm . . . well, it grows on you. But I need days to let it settle. The first day I could not stop thinking about all that I had left undone, notes unfinished, patients and trainees waiting, applications to be sent. Time usually feels so linear, yet never enough. Out here it's different—I can't explain it, it's inviting just to be. I have this feeling also in the mountains. It gives me peace.

Caroline smiles.

– It takes time to accept the invitation, doesn't it? To let yourself slow down without feeling like you're falling behind.

– More time than I want to admit. When I do, it feels like breathing again, like something is shifting, Karl Erik replies while still gazing at the horizon.

– Yes, Caroline says abruptly. I know what you mean. It's funny, though—sometimes I feel like the silence makes all the noise in my head change, like it amplifies everything. My thoughts don't speed up exactly—it's more like time thickens. It stretches wide but also pulls tight. There's this contrast— between stillness and speed, presence and focus. As if the quiet sharpens everything, and suddenly there's no escaping it. It's not slower—it's fuller.

Karl Erik sits down and takes a deep breath,

– I love the sensation when the heart just beats a tiny fraction slower. It's why I come back to places like this. To step into that fullness, to let the noise shift and take shape. I think I've spent a lot of time trying to quiet the noise, instead of . . . well, sorting through it. It's not just the quiet I come for. It pulls me from everything else, the work, the demands and expectations. I think of why I started in medicine, what it felt like to be sure of what I was doing even not knowing. Now, that certainty is harder to find.

Caroline, slipping off her shoes and letting her bare feet touch the rough surface of the stone:

– I know what you mean. I think, for me, it was always the stories that pulled me in. People's lives, their messiness. But somewhere along the way, the stories started sounding like noise. Even in psychiatry, where stories should be central, I find myself caught between the theory, the tools available to me, and the reality I face.

Karl Erik, becoming engaged and gesticulating with his hands:

– Yes! Sometimes I feel like I'm losing the meaning of what I am trying to do. There are the tensions between teaching and learning, between my research and clinical practice, but much more so between the systems and people. Between the technical solutions and care. I often feel like a stranger in many worlds, never belonging to any.

Caroline, nodding while letting her toes brush the cold water:

– And between disciplines that are supposed to work together but feel worlds apart. Psychiatry and infectious disease medicine couldn't be more different in some ways. And yet, I think we're both dealing with some of the same things. The noise, the gaps—the distance between what we're told medicine should be and what it feels like in practice.

Karl Erik, closing his eyes:

– Everyone is so busy keeping up that no one stops to ask why. Why we practise the way we do? Why we teach the way we do? Why we lead the way we do? Even why we chose this path in the first place?

Caroline, nodding and dipping her toes deeper into the water:

– Maybe it's not just about questioning the purpose. Maybe we also need to question the assumptions beneath it? Why do we assume efficiency should always come first? Why do we treat standardization as the ultimate goal—in patient care, in clinical decision making, in medical education?

Karl Erik, moving, showing his uneasiness:

– Well, I agree to a certain extent. I am, however, very humble towards the need for resource efficiency and the fair allocation of resources in public healthcare systems, like the ones we work in. We cannot turn a blind eye to that.

Caroline, turning her head:

> – Maybe. But we need to ask whose goals we are responding to. We talk about progress, but whose progress are we really serving. The patients'? Ours? The system's?

Karl Erik, taking a deep breath:

> – You are absolutely right, what patient-centred healthcare actually means in everyday clinical practice, from the time the patient enters the hospital to the point when they leave, is surprisingly complex and unclear, I think. Or maybe it is rather simple. The moment you lift your head, look, see, listen— then you are patient-centred. Simple, and remarkably difficult sometimes.

Caroline, raising her voice:

> – Hm, I need to ask: I noticed your puzzled and a bit unsure gaze today. During parts of the sessions before lunch?

Karl Erik, smiling:

> – You mean the sessions on the workload and all that? Well, yes, there are long hours, unrelenting pressure, and never enough time. There is exhaustion, yes. But I don't feel it to the extent that it was felt by some in the room today. And quite frankly it's not new to me; I hear it from colleagues as well. It puzzles me: Is something strange or wrong with me? I wonder if we, as young doctors, as a group, are not humble enough to the various stages of learning, of growing into a profession. It does hurt. Sometimes I think it needs to hurt . . . I am not saying that all the work overload is OK, and many parts of the system for taking care of doctors in training can be better. But I am not sure if I buy into the whole gloomy picture that is being painted.

Caroline, a bit surprised:

> – I do think I know what you mean. However, I was a bit surprised with some of the more experienced colleagues, what they were thinking when they heard the stories of burnout, pressure, and endless hours. They were surprisingly quiet? As if they were thinking back, being reminded of their

old age and how they themselves had forgotten the struggles they had to go through, maybe even thinking about how much harder it was before? Even longer shifts? Even more patients to handle per doctor? Even more responsibility? Maybe they are just tired of hearing it? I keep imagining they are all thinking "it was much harder in my time!" But they don't say it out loud. Maybe because they know it doesn't bridge the gap.

Karl Erik, nodding:

– To speak of it would mean to confront experiences they may want to keep buried. And it is more complicated than that; it's a distance between understanding and not. I feel that distance too, to be honest. I hear what my colleagues are saying; I hear and sometimes also recognise their stories, but I have to be honest, they don't fully resonate with me. It makes me feel uneasy: Where do I fit in the puzzle? I am sure there is an insight there, I just haven't discovered it yet.

Caroline, turning her head, raising an eyebrow:

– Pain demands attention; there is often little room for critique. There is a tension between pain and reflection, between questions and assumptions. In the burnout, in the despair, it's a lot of circling around, using rigid interpretations to make it manageable. If someone is struggling, we answer, almost as a reflex—we need more mindfulness! Or better work–life balance! Or we reduce it to a critique of rigid institutions or lack of resources—as if it's all the fault of the system. There is a gap between what the work is and what we imagine it to be.

Karl Erik takes a deep breath, leaving a short pause in the discussion:

– We try to do it all. Medicine is art and science, they both have their place, deeply intertwined, but also different. Losing one part, however, leads to lack of meaning. The art part is so much, it's about stories, about relationships, about biography. The science part is about precision and protocols, it's much more action-oriented. I often find myself lost between two cultures, as described by CP Snow (1959). But we have to stop re-creating this division. Of course, when I get sick, I want a doctor with sound biomedical knowledge, but that is certainly not enough. I also want a doctor who sees me, listens to my story, my values, and my ideas—I am not prepared for a medical practice which is guideline-obese and only sees me as an object to be risk-stratified.

Caroline adjusts her position, laughs, and turns her head towards Karl Erik:

– Guideline-obese, that's a new one! But I think it's not only between the disciplines there is this division, the "two worlds" so to say. It's between colleagues and generations. I sense that the human side is slipping further away, buried under all the guidelines and all the advancements. And I am not saying the innovations are wrong or bad. We can't ignore them—but they often come with a cost. The closer we get to perfecting the technical, the harder it becomes to hold onto the relational. To balance the art and the science without one overwhelming the other is very difficult.

Karl Erik nods while straightening his back as if he has something important to say:

– And it is in that balance I find the wisdom from so many colleagues. I am very lucky to have many of those at my hospital. I am very encouraged and find great motivation in how my colleagues give personalised medicine or patient-oriented medicine real meaning. It is the balancing of what we know from all the advanced studies with what fits for the person in front of them. Having colleagues like that is very formative when you start a professional career and of course also later. I am often encouraged by seeing how older colleagues live comfortably in the grey zones, the zones where we don't know for sure. To be frank, I think the science part has led to great advancement, but that it is often also overselling the story—which in itself can cause a great deal of harm.

Karl Erik pauses for a moment, a grimace on his face, clearly indicating his discomfort:

– Do you think there is a gender issue? It is such a difficult question, but I feel it is there, under the surface. I notice that many of my female colleagues seem to carry a different mental load. They seem less confident at times, or maybe it is the socialization of doubt. And on the other side they are less concerned with addressing their concern. Does this resonate with you, or am I too simplistic?

Caroline leans forward, pauses, and stutters the first words:

> – I don't think it sounds wrong, but it is clearly more complicated. Women are often socialised as caregivers, to take responsibility for work and people around them. I think that it is often a great strength, but in a field that becomes less relational and more technical—it can take a bigger toll on them. The system doesn't always help; there is an endless focus on efficiency, technical skill, and decisiveness. All this is important, but it leaves less room for the relational and what makes the work human.

Karl Erik nods softly. There is discomfort in his face:

> – And this strain of always feeling you have to prove yourself, to balance everything perfectly in all parts of life—home and work. It's not that men don't feel it too, but maybe it is different for us. It is a big loss for us all, men and women, when the relational is sidelined. The whole system suffers. We lose direction, we lose fundamental meaning.

Caroline pauses, her voice quiet:

> – And it is not just about us, it's about the patients, the society we live in, and the expectations. Medicine has shifted from care to facilitation, from guiding to the presenting of options. We are not seen any more as healers, we are facilitators. That changes the dynamic profoundly. Autonomy is essential; it empowers the patients, and nobody wants to move away from that. But it is also complicated. We have become translators of guidelines, mediators between the possible and the guidelines. It is not just about offering choices, but helping patients make sense of them. That requires engagement, time, presence, and deep listening.

Karl Erik leans back, exhaling slowly:

> – Yes. I think you are completely right. And in this process you are, as a doctor, not only on the giving end of it, you are also at the receiving end. I think that is such a meaningful dimension of our profession. You have to be willing to learn from your patients and colleagues. That is not easy when you are supposed to be so perfect in all aspects. It opens you up to vulnerability and therefore requires humility about not having all the answers. Although by some regarded as weakness, I have always

found that in talking to patients and relatives, opening up about the unknown and about the limits of medicine gives them comfort. Being a doctor is not about knowing everything—nobody does. It's about knowing enough—and knowing what matters. That is of course hard to do, but I see this in some of my senior colleagues. They show me what phronesis actually means. They have the ability to see the bigger picture without losing the human connection. It sounds almost paternalistic and arrogant, but it is not. They know when to act and when to stop or wait. They carry themselves with a quiet confidence, an assuredness that puts everyone at ease.

Caroline, smiling and engaged:

– I have colleagues like that too. It's like they hold the space, isn't it? For everyone, for the patients, for colleagues. They're not treating disease or symptoms, they're holding situations. They are not afraid of the uncertainty, the complexity. And the key, I think, is that they see it as part of their work, not something to overcome, but something to engage with. It makes me think of a colleague when I was at the beginning of my hospital training. He is not the loudest, doesn't speak in big letters, but the way he works was inspiring. Always humble, always collaborative, always grounded. I went to him with a case I thought, quite frankly, I had completely messed up. But instead, he said, let's figure it out together. We dissected the case together, he never taught me, he guided me, and together, we figured it out. He showed that it is about the approach, it's OK not to know it all. He taught me how to stay calm in uncertainty. I carry this with me every day. I use that not only as a doctor but also when I train others, how I create space for them, trying to avoid filling the gaps for them. Having experiences like that in the beginning is important.

Karl Erik, smiling, with a calm voice:

– And it stayed with you because it was not only about solving the problem, but how to think, of relating. He showed what it means to practise with humility and presence. That's phronesis. It's about showing up, being willing to learn, and helping others to do the same. It's not about perfection. Or maybe that's what it is—perfection!

Caroline laughs:

> – The question is though, how do you think this kind of practical wisdom comes into being? Is it possible to pass it on? Our senior colleagues trained as clinicians in a different world under different conditions. The practices, the structures, the relationships were different then. I wonder if the conditions that nurtured the wisdom we are discussing are disappearing.

Karl Erik, his eyes now firm:

> – It is not something you can teach in a lecture hall or assess at an exam. It's not something you can tick off in a box or a procedural list. I often find myself sad because I feel I am not able to offer the wisdom I have learnt to younger colleagues.

Caroline pauses, a question in her voice:

> – We've talked about responsibility, engagement, and reciprocity—underneath all of it there is this nagging question, what is the meaning of it all? What is the purpose now, when the nature of medicine has shifted so much?

Karl Erik, contemplative:

> – It's a question we avoid too often. We talk about patient satisfaction, outcome, adherence to guidelines—but we very rarely take a step back to ask what is it all for? Medicine has become so fragmented, so mechanised. I quite often have to stop myself and think what is the meaning of this? We focus on what we are doing, but seem sometimes to lose sight of why we are doing it. And maybe that's why we see so much burnout and frustration in young colleagues. It is not just the workload, it's the lack of grounding.

Caroline, looking down at her hands, leaning forward:

> – They're . . . well, we're all . . . working in a space where the old ideals don't fit and new ones have to fully emerge. We're caught in this in-between place, trying to hold on to something meaningful from the past, while adapting to a future we can't quite see the dimensions of yet. And if we are losing what matters, what we just talked about, the art and the wisdom, how do we nurture it anew? What would it take to

make space for this wisdom to emerge in the medical reality we inhabit today?

Karl Erik looks up and speaks towards the sea:

– I think part of the key is the acknowledgment that it will never be perfect. And believing in ourselves, that we can make a difference for the patients and our colleagues, even with all the constraints. It's not easy, I admit, and maybe we need many more moments like these, to pause, to ask not only what, but why?

Caroline, smiling and turning her face:

– And to ask who we are doing it with? Maybe that's what reciprocity means—a shared process of making meaning, we can't do it alone. Whether it's with patients, students, or colleagues.

Karl Erik stands up, brushes his hair, and gazes at the horizon:

– And it's about trust, daring to trust that even in the imperfection we are contributing to something larger. These small moments, which I feel the system overlooks or at least doesn't give enough attention to, that's where the real work happens. It's not a perfect system, it never was, and it will never be. But we are also the system, we can shape it, we can transform it, in everything we do.

Caroline smiles:

– Then let's start there, with these small, everyday, imperfect moments. And now, let's get back to the noise.

Reference

Snow, C. P. (1959). *The two cultures and the scientific revolution.* Cambridge University Press.

14

Wisdom in Medical Practice

J. Donald Boudreau

Introduction

These days, many physicians and clinical teachers are lusty participants in or engaged witnesses to the incorporation of artificial intelligence (AI) in healthcare. The developments are striking. A recent study has confirmed that large language models, such as ChatGPT, can engage with patients in human-like communication—to the point of replicating conversations with empathic overtones. The potential of AI to assist healthcare professionals with the entire gamut of professional obligations, from the mundane and routine (such as disinfecting bedpans), to the sophisticated and venerable (such as initiating cancer treatments), and everything in between, is remarkable.

Promises made on behalf of AI can seem boundless. Exactly in what forms this new technology will end up contributing to overall doctor and patient experiences have yet to be clarified. As with most innovations initially touted to be wonderous in scope and quality, limitations will surely become apparent, and the waves of untrammelled enthusiasm will be tempered. While we wait for the pendulum to find a congenial midpoint between endorsement and restraint, these developments remind us of the need to be clear as to what are the essential qualities of doctoring and to nurture those that are impervious to technological replication or improvement.

Could a robot be assembled to resemble a sapient creature and to assume the bulk of clinical responsibilities? Are there tasks that cannot be replicated by

DOI: 10.1201/9781003593294-14

social robots? Reflecting on the distinctions between the nature of humans and robots, while foregrounding the *sine qua non* of clinical care, has the potential to reveal the "indispensable stuff" of medicine. I will attempt to trace out some of those contours. I will argue that there is overlap between those ingredients and features of practical wisdom.

Setting the Scene with a Clinical Case

I begin my exploration by considering a clinical scenario and imagining how two versions of it might unfold. Version I will have a patient and a robotic clinician as interlocutors. Version II will present the same patient, but with an "in-the-flesh" physician. The second version will be described in greater detail. This is not because I desire, from the get-go, to paint the first version in an unfair light. It simply reflects the fact that I am much more familiar with the setting and protagonists in the second version. Our imagined clinical robot is labelled MDx-CY2, and the name of our imagined physician is Dr Arthur Seguro.

Patient

Jesse Roja is a 56-year-old man, the owner of a bookstore. Jesse has developed a health problem. He has seen blood in his ejaculate on three occasions in the past eight months. He is worried about cancer and has also wondered about venereal diseases. He is baffled as to how to tell his partner about it. The situation finds him petrified and, to some extent, emotionally paralyzed.

For most generalist physicians, the experience of having to deal with this symptom in the clinic would likely be bewildering, perhaps even intimidating. Haematospermia is not a symptom in the same league as haematuria, haematochezia, or haemoptysis. The latter are classic fare in "introduction to clinical medicine" type courses. Those symptoms are ensconced in the standard repertoire of the "functional enquiry" the card deck of prompts with which junior medical students arm themselves as they learn the tricks of the trade. In the interview of a patient, they are deployed in a manner that is not unlike a police interrogation:

- *Is your urine ever pink or red?*
- *Have you seen blood in your stool? If so, is it on the outside or mixed in?*
- *Is the stool black?*

- *Have you vomited blood?*
- *Is the phlegm blood-tinged? Can you estimate, in teaspoons, how much blood you coughed up in the past 24 hours?*
- *Do you have nosebleeds, bleeding gums?*
- *Do you take blood thinners?*

These rote questions roll off the tongue as automatically as a knee jerks in response to a tap on the patellar tendon. For the physician, there is a familiarity with the clinical scripts which these symptoms evoke: Urinary infection, haemorrhoids, gastric ulcers, pneumococcal pneumonia, bronchogenic carcinoma, and the like. Blood in the sperm, however, is an entirely different kettle of fish. For one thing, it conjures up sex. It can summon various sexually acquired diseases to the differential diagnosis. For patient and physician alike, these subjects are frequently embarrassing or taboo. Second, because the ejaculate represents a sort of passport for procreation, a blighted specimen may be interpreted as an affront to promise and potential. Third, it is an unusual and foreign symptom. It is not showcased in popular art forms; it has no thespian counterparts to the consumptive heroines in *La Traviata* or *La Bohème*, women who are seen coughing in a handkerchief and then surreptitiously folding it in order to conceal specs of blood. There is no companion to the opening scene of the film, *The Decline of the American Empire*, where a protagonist is startled to see his urinary stream rendering the water in a toilet bowl beet red. Haematospermia has seldom made an appearance in mainstream cultural representations. Fourth, there is something visually arresting with the colour red superimposed on a background of creamy white. No, that symptom is unlike others. It is obscure. It is "messy." It is not amenable to problem solving through conveniently available clinical practice guidelines. It is entangled in thick layers of meanings. Unravelling this requires clinical knowledge and discernment. One must tread carefully. It demands exquisite sensibility, sympathy, and an interlocutor who is an attentive listener, especially alert to the hidden messages revealed in language and paralanguage.

Clinical Encounter—Version I (Intervention by a Robot)

MDx-CY2 is impressive. It is a humanoid robot. It is 175 cm in height; androgynous; has a lifelike human face capable of expressions and automated eye contact; a 2D camera, several directional microphones and speakers, touch sensors; and the ability to grasp objects, walk, and squat. It comes equipped with superb clinically relevant tools, including:

- The most recent version of a large language model—enabling focused medical history taking and its documentation using adaptable templates.
- Avant-garde sensors—allowing for the gathering of biodata such as blood pressure, pulse, core temperature, body mass index (BMI), oxygen saturation, transcutaneous bilirubinometry, transcutaneous haemoglobin, and plasma glucose measurements; echographic estimates of left ventricular end-diastolic pressure; ultrasound measurements of hepatic, splenic, aortic, and uterine dimensions; dermatoscopic-guided comprehensive survey of the skin for malignancy; transient elastography screening for liver fibrosis; and numerous other optional applications that can ferret out specific medical conditions.
- Platforms for clinical decision making, supported by decision tree algorithms, clinical practice guidelines, and extensive databases on disease prevalence in many different nations and communities— resulting in estimates of prior probabilities and, using sophisticated statistics and the sequential application of Bayes theorem, the ability to calculate robust likelihood ratios and conditional probabilities.
- A humongous database, with unfettered access to PubMed Central and UpToDate—enabling the generation of impressive differential diagnoses in appropriate order of likelihood.
- Drug decision support and drug interaction databases—facilitating sophisticated and evidence-based treatment recommendations.
- AI—endowing it with the ability to learn new strategies and new tasks.

In short, the components constitutive of MDx-CY2 render it a realistic, interactive, clinically skilful, and competent diagnostician. It is able to propose a defensible and appropriate treatment plan.

MDx-CY2 encounters Mr Roja in a "Comprehensive and Integrated Well-Being Institute" affiliated with an academic health centre. The consultation room where they meet is quiet, well lit, beige, windowless, and comfortable. It is well appointed with sophisticated ancillary clinical equipment. Following an orientation to the process and a request for the patient to complete a standard "description of current concern" form and to sign a consent, the robot proceeds with an interview, examination, and analysis of the issue at hand.

Mr Roja experiences the interaction as laconic and unhurried, tinged with an air of a deliberate and no-nonsense seriousness. The robot considers benign and malignant conditions, favouring the former. It points out the lack of constitutional symptoms such as weight loss and fever, the absence of any evidence for a bleeding diathesis, and notes that there have been periods of several months where the client has been completely asymptomatic. It closes the encounter by providing relevant information, supplemented by reading materials specifically designed for patient consumption, and by recommending a series of investigations, including blood tests and a transurethral ultrasound. It offers to perform these tests in a "Male Reproductive and Sexual Health" multiservice centre, located within the same "institute." The centre has a good reputation for effective and efficient client service. It is staffed by a team of urologists, endocrinologists, and psychologists, and they are all equipped with robotic assistants.

Clinical Encounter—Version II (Intervention by an "In-the-Flesh" Physician)

Dr Arthur Seguro, a general practitioner, is a mid-career physician who has been in practice, working in a private clinic, for approximately 20 years. Over the years, his practice has gravitated towards adult medicine. He no longer takes care of children, nor is he involved in anaesthesia, surgery, or critical care. His patient population is highly varied in terms of age, gender, socioeconomic status, and ethnicity. This diversity brings him much professional satisfaction. He has cultivated an interest in infectious diseases and works at a tropical medicine clinic and at a clinic specializing in sexually transmitted diseases once per week in each of these specialty clinics. He has amassed a small cadre of patients who are avid travellers and another of male patients who have sexual and/or romantic attraction to other males. He is quite attuned to disease prevention and is frequently asked to prescribe vaccines, malaria prophylaxis, and the pre-exposure prophylaxis (PrEP) option for HIV. He is an amiable and garrulous individual who has access to a wealth of consultants from many disciplines and to several well-established corridors of healthcare service in the community.

Dr Seguro receives Mr Roja at his general clinic. The consultation room looks a bit dated with furniture, examining table, and equipment that are rough around the edges. The wall is a salmon colour, somewhat faded. There are pictures of dogs on the wall and on the desk: An Australian Shepherd, a Golden Retriever, and a pair of long-haired Dachshunds. It transpires to be a particularly chaotic day for the encounter. Following introductions and a smidgen of small talk, Dr Seguro asks how he can be of help. Mr Roja gets right to the point: *"This is a little embarrassing. I have blood in my sperm."* Dr Seguro continues with the history, trying not to interrupt too often, but because he is late in his appointments, he is not as "all ears" as he would like to be.

[Dr AS's inner voice: *It is so busy; I've got to rush.*]

[Dr AS's body: Edgy.]

He slides into his *"approach to bleeding from any orifice"* script, focusing on (i) bleeding from additional sites (nose, gums, stool, urine); (ii) family history of bleeding; (iii) use of aspirin, anticoagulants, or antiplatelets; (iv) easy bruisability. This is immediately followed by a series of questions concerning life-threatening illness and conditions that must not be missed, such as leukaemia or cancer: "Has there been any weight loss, lethargy, fever, recent infections, bone pain?" Because of time constraints, and against his better judgement, Dr Seguro coasts towards ending the interview a bit prematurely; he switches to the genitourinary functional enquiry. Prostate problems loom in his mind; he thinks of chronic prostatitis, prostatic cancer, tuberculosis: "Is there pain or burning on peeing; when you have the urge to go, does it feel urgent; how strong is the urinary stream; any episodes of incontinence; how many times do you wake up to pee?"

[Dr AS's inner voice: *There are other questions I need to ask. I am not sure which ones. This is my first time with this symptom. Why did TB cross my mind? Weird. Think of the basics . . . like trauma. Oh my, perhaps this guy uses sex toys that have traumatized his urethra and that explains why he has blood intermittently in his sperm. But I can't go there . . . yet. Park that thought.*]

He now goes on to a brief and focused physical examination. He takes the pulse and blood pressure. He looks at the conjunctiva for pallor, intentionally putting his right hand on the patient's left shoulder, an unconscious reflex aimed at reassurance and showing sympathy and concern. He takes a cursory listen to the precordium, almost like an automaton—going through the motion—then asks the patient to lie down and palpates the abdomen. He senses that the patient is ticklish and adjusts his movements.

He puts on gloves, inspects the genitals. He asks if the patient can turn to his left side to do a digital rectal exam. He feels the prostate, summoning the memory of his fingertips, mentally trying to compare its size, symmetry, and texture with the hundreds of prostates he has palpated over the 30 or so years since he started medical school.

[Dr AS's inner voice: *This man is clean, well nourished, cooperative, intelligent, coherent. I see no rash. No tattoos. No penile discharge. I think there may be more than meets the eye. I need to deal with this in another visit.*]

[Dr AS's body: His gut or a sixth sense tells him that the patient is frightened.]

He concludes the meeting: *"Mr Roja, I don't know a lot about blood in the ejaculate. From my recollection as a medical student, it is generally a benign condition that goes away by itself. I need to read more about it. I will need to see you again to continue our conversation and for me to get to know you better. In the meanwhile, I would like to do an analysis of the urine, including a culture, and some routine blood test. Could we see each other for a follow-up in two weeks?"*

[Dr AS's inner voice: *I hope I have allayed some of his fears. I avoided mentioning the PSA blood test. Was that a mistake? Perhaps he picked up on this omission. I would not be surprised that he has read about haematospermia, prostate cancer, screening for prostate cancer, and much more on the internet.*

Oh my. What a morning.

What's next!]

An Analysis of the Case and What It Reveals about Characteristics of Medical Practice

The purpose of the case was not to initiate a discussion on the potential contributions of data and computer sciences or on the emerging role of technological innovations, such as AI, to medical practice. It is not meant as a springboard to question, analyse, endorse, criticize, predict, or portray what the future may hold for social robots in the clinic. Rather, in setting the scene with versions I and II, I am inviting the reader to compare the two imaginary encounters and, in doing so, to contemplate what might be the good and the right ingredients of clinical practice. It will be useful for the reader to try to envisage where a social robot might succeed or prevail and where it might struggle, find itself out in left field, or miss the boat entirely as it responds to the patient.

There are many contrasting features between the two encounters. The most striking—and this should be evident from how I structured and represented the clinical scenarios—is the absence of metacognition in version I and its presence in Version II. Dr Seguro engages in active contemplation in a special space where beliefs are examined; truth claims, intentions, and motivations enter into deliberation; emotions and cognition are intertwined, i.e., where he thinks his emotions and feels his thoughts; and, where meaning making occurs. The inner voice reverberates and commands attention. Dr Seguro's body also communicates with him; in some instances, the seat of the message, metaphorically speaking, is the gut. These are aspects of conscious and non-conscious reflection (Schei et al., 2019).

MDx-CY2 has not been assembled with templates that are aligned with the special space described earlier. MDx-CY2 can evaluate its behaviours based on the mental models with which it has been programmed. Through an algorithmic processing of alignment of a particular action with mental models, the social robot can self-evaluate. However, it has no access to the foundational meanings of the core beliefs and values encapsulated in those mental models. Also, it holds no currency in affective domains. The robot's capabilities in this regard represent an impoverished version of reflection, as is generally conceived of in the humanities. This is an important observation because reflection is a core feature of medical practice. It is a duty of the medical teacher to support and nurture reflection. William Osler (1950) expressed this obligation as follows: "Let us emancipate the student and give him (them) time and opportunity for the cultivation of his (their) mind, so that in his (their) pupilage he (they) shall not be a puppet in the hands of others, but rather a self-relying and reflecting being."

So, version I is devoid of a reflective capability. And there are no embodied perceptions. These are two important aspects of clinical care. I suggest that they are critical ingredients in the cornucopia of medicine's "indispensable stuff." They are also features of wise practices. Let us now discuss additional differences between the first and second versions of that hypothetical clinical interaction.

Dr Seguro is influenced by the socio-material conditions in which he finds himself. For example, a malfunctioning air-conditioning unit will result in a rise in ambient temperature; this may negatively impact his performance. His physiological state will almost certainly have an outsized influence. Perhaps he is tired due to a poor night's sleep or is jittery and tremulous because of having had too much coffee that morning or having imbibed excessively the night before. Perhaps his tennis elbow or allergies are particularly bothersome that day. Perhaps he is hungry. Factors as seemingly humdrum as date—time of day, day of the week, month, season—can be relevant. While temporal proximity to a vacation, birthday, or dental appointment is immaterial to MDx-CY2, these sorts of contextual factors can impinge on a person's ability to focus. In contrast, the robot is impervious to such considerations.

Dr AS's decision making may be subject to a multitude of cognitive biases to which MDx-CY2 is immune. For example, in the case of Jesse Roja, Dr Seguro may have landed on a provisional diagnosis of prostatic tuberculosis in part because he was involved with a case one month ago. This is called the availability heuristic; humans tend to think that things which happened recently will happen again. Or, he may fall prey to an unfortunate train of thought propelled by prejudices. For example, he may have observed certain effeminate gestures in Mr Roja and have jumped to the conclusion that Mr Roja is a gay man. Due to potent personal biases, he may then have linked gay-ness with licentious-ness and have arrived at a tentative diagnosis of a sexually transmitted disease. As well as demonstrating prejudgement this also illustrates features of an attribution error, i.e., where one overemphasizes the importance of dispositions or internal (in this instance, effeminate behaviours) over external factors.

In considering these differences, one may conclude that the robot possesses staggering advantages. To be shielded from things like sleep deprivation or hunger and to be exempt from cognitive biases and prejudice is surely a useful attribute. But, at the same time, such characteristics are not always liabilities—not invariably. The inability to feel hunger, thirst, sexual urges, surprise, curiosity, happiness, grief, pain, pity, pride, love, fear, admiration, disgust, and myriad other human emotions and to experience manifestations of suffering must surely represent an obdurate barrier to a robot's potential for compassionate understanding and empathic responses. Even with regard to cognition, a domain in which the merits of robotics are taken for granted, one could argue that our imagined physician's musing on the possibility of prostatic tuberculosis might end up being the educated guess or a shot in the dark that amounts to a stroke of genius. His diagnostic leap could represent the abductive reasoning and creative impulses that often are markers of clinical acumen.

It is self-evident that humans and robots are not made from the same cloth. Sinews have little in common with semiconductor chips. The idea that clinicians can be affected by features such as the timing of an encounter with a patient because of links to meaningful aspects in their lived experiences (e.g., the Shabbat, Lent, Ramadan) or the realization that personal functioning can easily become a prisoner to the frailties of the human condition (e.g., inability to sit on a chair due to the intrusion of lowly haemorrhoids) reminds us of that gaping dissimilarity.

Another critical difference is the relationship with certainty. Dr Seguro's professional life is awash in uncertainty and ambiguity; his clinical world is one of unavoidable contingencies, i.e., events or circumstances that cannot be predicted with certainty. This essential and ineluctable characteristic of medical practice was expressed in a recently published empirical study on the clinical practices of exemplary physicians (Boudreau et al., 2024). A participant in that research, a paediatric surgeon, described his practice as one "where the numbers zero and one hundred do not exist." Indeed, it is rare in medicine that an outcome can be captured with the assuredness that this will *never* happen or will *always* happen. In contrast, our imagined robot, as the American colloquial expression goes, "pays no nevermind" to uncertainty.

This preamble revealed some of the features that make medical practice unique, frustrating, and rewarding. Our imagined robot MDx-CY2 served as a foil. It permitted us to emphasize how the world of medical practice cannot be completely understood with the predictability and generalizability of scientific reasoning or the routinized and algorithmized constitutional makeup of a social robot. In short, medicine is an endeavour that requires practical knowledge, practical skills, and practical know-how. The clinician's personal dispositions, approaches to seeing and perceiving, habits of working, manners of interacting with others, modes of thinking, and ways of conceiving the means and ends of clinical actions are all determined and moulded by its practical nature. These dispositions, modes, ways, habits, and manners must be responsive to the types of demands, opportunities, and constraints we have just considered using the heuristic of an imagined clinical scenario.

Characteristics of a "Wise" Clinician—In the Practical Sense

An exemplary and consummate clinician is one who, through years of experience, accompanied by guided reflection and often supported by wise mentors, has acquired wisdom of a practical nature.

It is beyond the remit of this chapter to do a deep dive in the concept of practical wisdom, to trace its time-honoured pedigree, to offer fulsome descriptions of its manifestations in all human domains, or to do justice to contemporary research in the domain. Remarkable insights on its nature and how it contrasts with other modes of human thought and action are to be found in the philosophical literature, notably in Aristotle's *Nicomachean Ethics*. Aristotle refers to the concept as *phronesis*. Numerous scholars, notably Martin Heidegger, Hans-Georg Gadamer, Alasdair MacIntyre, Joseph Dunne, and Edmund Pellegrino, have refined and enriched our collective understanding of practical wisdom. My aims for this chapter are modest. It will serve as a basic introduction while underlining how it differs from and complements technical and scientific modes of reasoning.

I realize that, in launching this discussion I may have inadvertently set up a tug-of-war between a social robot and an "in-the-flesh" physician. It was not my intention to create a conflictual situation. It is much too facile to brandish science (symbolized by MDx-CY2) as rational, objective, value neutral, and computational and, in contrast, to showcase the humanities (embodied by Dr Seguro) as relational, subjective, affective, and multidimensional. I find that the script of irreconcilable dichotomies, such as art and science or psyche and soma, has been overplayed. This is a zero-sum game that should be avoided. Contemporary medicine requires technology; practising medicine without it would be a dishonest, desiccated, and futile endeavour. The point I wish to make is that medicine is a polyglot; it relies on many perspectives. Therefore, it is advisable to remind ourselves of all the languages, voices, and worldviews that are constitutive of medicine.

In collaboration with talented and esteemed colleagues, I have written about practical wisdom in the context of medicine. An opinion piece, entitled "Medical Wisdom" endorsed a perspective previously advanced by Katherine Montgomery Hunter (2005) that clinical thinking includes two complementary movements, generalization and particularization. We argued that the process of generalization has been well conceptualized while particularization has been much less so. Grounded in the conviction that medical practice is focused on an "N of '1'," that is, a unique and singular patient, we advocated for an increased focus on particularization. To that end, we described features of an intellectual framing leading to and favouring particularization (Boudreau & Cassell, 2021). We suggested that interpretations of the narrative structures of a clinical case are effective at rendering visible, in rich and thick 3D panoramas, the particularities of a case. Narrative competence constitutes some of the "right stuff" of medicine.

To further delineate the contours of practical wisdom in medicine, we followed our theoretical exploration with empirical studies. We recently examined the practices of a small cadre of exemplary physicians (Saraga et al., 2019). We found that their medical practices could be broadly described as "engagement" in the clinical situation. The facets of this engagement included the ability of a clinician: to create a space/time bubble within which the clinical encounter unfolds; to trespass boundaries or break rules for compassionate reasons; to conceive of their work as "doing an honest job"; to assume responsibility and be accountable. Our findings pointed to practical wisdom as a central dimension. A secondary analysis of the data revealed the following characteristics: wise physicians have a particular character (ethos) and clinical know-how (habitus); they encounter their patients with attentiveness; they utilize modes of reasoning which help them cope with complexity and uncertainty; and they refer to certain aspects of their practice which have an elusive or *je ne sais quoi* quality (e.g., such as relying on gut feelings). We referred to this constellation of characteristics as "clinical phronesis." We have been cautious in not claiming that the qualities of practical wisdom we have excavated are universally present across all communities or cultures or that they are timeless and changeless. Nonetheless, we hope that such qualities will remain at the centre of our collective professional attention. A recent review of the literature has summarized the traditional and emergent characteristics of phronesis in medicine (Jameel, 2025). It is gratifying to see how enthusiastically phronesis has been taken up in contemporary health sciences education research.

The understanding of clinical work that emerged from our research "is at odds with a portrayal of medicine that presents a detached physician, equipped with the knowledge of bioscience and trained in pre-defined competencies, who arrives at a diagnosis and selects therapies following algorithmic practice guidelines" (Boudreau et al., 2024). This account of wise medical practice may act as a bulwark against a portrayal of medicine that invites clinicians to be *superseded* by social robots such as MDx-CY2. Having said this, I would not want to leave the reader with the impression that clinical phronesis is a sort of an antidote to a practice gone awry or an agentic force destined to emancipate us from the continued encroachment of technology. Technology is indispensable for modern medicine. Social robots have a role to play in the sick room, for example, in an *assistive* function. They need to be embraced and integrated prudentially and with humility. It is my hope that understanding the nature of phronesis will help teachers and their students complement their scientific knowledge, technical skills, and innate humanistic dispositions with the valuable lessons taught to us by the lived examples of exemplary clinicians.

References

Boudreau, D., & Cassell, E. J. (2021). Medical wisdom. *Perspectives in Biology and Medicine, 64*(2), 251–270.

Boudreau, D., Wykretowicz, H., Kinsella, E. A., Fuks, A., & Saraga, M. (2024). Discovering clinical phronesis. *Medicine, Health Care and Philosophy*. https://link.springer.com/article/10.1007/s11019-024-10198-8

Hunter, K. M. (2005). *How doctors think: Clinical judgment and the practice of medicine.* Oxford University Press.

Jameel, S. Y. (2025). A critical interpretive literature review of phronesis in medicine. *Journal of Medicine and Philosophy, 50*(2), 104–116.

Osler, W. (1950). *Osler Aphorisms, from his bedside teachings and writings.* Henry Schuman, Inc. Retrieved June 30, 2024, from https://archive.org/stream/in.ernet.dli.2015.63933/2015.63933.Osler-Aphorisms-From-His-Bedside-Teachings-And-Writings_djvu.txt

Saraga, M., Boudreau, D., & Fuks, A. (2019). Engagement and practical wisdom in clinical practice: A phenomenological study. *Medicine, Health Care and Philosophy, 22*(1), 41–52.

Schei, E., Fuks, A., & Boudreau, D. (2019). Reflection in medical education: Intellectual humility, discovery and know-how. *Medicine, Health Care and Philosophy, 22*(2), 167–178.

15

Why I Run

Lizzie Wastnedge

It's 7 a.m. on a Thursday morning in November, and I am climbing steeply up Barrow, still barely awake, coming into consciousness incrementally with each sharp intake of breath. Keswick falls away behind me and is soon hidden in the early morning mist which sits heavily over Derwentwater. I crest the brow of the hill as the sun breaks the horizon, casting a soft glow over the hillside and illuminating the autumnal colours of the trees surrounding the lake. As I reach the summit, I too am bathed in golden rays, warm despite the frosty night still hard on the ground. For the first time in what feels like weeks, my face cracks into a genuine smile of pure joy—this is why I run.

Twelve hours earlier, I had just left work feeling exhausted. I am currently working as a junior doctor in Edinburgh, and the busy role, the shifts, the staffing shortages, all exacerbated by the pandemic, had finally become too much and I was entirely burnt out. I had one day off that week, prior to what would doubtlessly be a gruelling weekend. I knew that finishing work on Wednesday evening, sleeping in my van in Keswick, attempting to run 30 miles and then driving back to work three 13-hour shifts may, for some, seem close to lunacy. Yet, I also knew it was the only way I would get through the weekend, and as I stood on the ridge and watched the sunrise from behind the hills, I knew I had made the right decision.

The Abraham's Tea Round had been on my to-do list for a while. The route takes in all the summits visible from the café in George Fisher's outdoor shop and with 12,000 feet of ascent over 30 miles, the run is no mean feat. My recent shift pattern had taken a toll on my fitness, and as I started climbing, my chest felt tight. I hadn't been sleeping and felt physically and

DOI: 10.1201/9781003593294-15

mentally exhausted. When I set out it seemed unlikely I would succeed in completing the whole round that day, but the forecast was perfect and as the sun burnt off the last of the morning fog, I felt confident I would have a lovely day—irrespective of how far I managed.

From the top of Barrow I drop down and then climb steeply to reach the ridge of the Coledale horseshoe. As I warm up I find a steady rhythm and begin to relax into a comfortable pace, thinking of nothing more than my breathing and the pounding of my feet. Finally, after a week of tense, anxious ruminating I am grounded and my mind feels still and peaceful.

I came to running from climbing. I moved up to Edinburgh for medical school, joined the mountaineering club, and was soon spending every weekend in the hills. I found as I grew in confidence moving in the mountains, running felt like a natural progression. Over time, it became something I not only loved but depended on. I first felt really low at university. I had learned about "depression" and "anxiety" during my studies; however, the textbook excerpts I had memorized for exams seemed to bear little relation to the sheer weight of desolation which engulfed me. The stultifying and all-encompassing sense of acute yet deadening despair rendered everything around me dulled and flattened. I felt like I saw the world through a hazy fog, unable to glean true enjoyment or pleasure from anything. I talked to very few people about how bad things were—feeling ashamed and uncertain how my friends would react, yet maintaining a front of normality was exhausting and further deepened my sense of isolation. In running, however, I found a release. The simple act of placing each foot in front of the other felt meditative and centring. As my fitness improved, maintaining and pushing myself further gave me a reason to keep going each day. Gradually the clouds lifted.

I round the Coledale horseshoe in good time. Knowing how tired I was, I had worked out a couple of escape routes to cut the round short; however, I pass the first of these feeling fresh. I make good time down from Grisedale Pike, and as I reach Whiteless Pike the sun is high in the cloudless sky and I feel refreshed and strong. I race down the steep grassy slope towards Buttermere, allowing gravity to carry me down the hill, enjoying the dance between rocks and tussocks, descending as fast as I dare on the tightrope balance between speed and loss of control. I reach Buttermere and another possible route home but leave this behind with little thought and wend my way between Buttermere and Crummock Water to start the steep climb up Red Pike. As I ascend my heart pounds almost painfully in my chest and my calves burn. Each breath in is a gasp yet I push harder and move faster, forcing myself to my physical limit. As I exhaust myself physically, I find my mind able to relax and I begin to mull over some of the challenging cases I had encountered in the preceding weeks—the angry patients frustrated by long waiting lists, the broken souls worn down by systematic hardships, the deaths (both expected and untimely), the people I told they would live, the people I told they would die. When I applied for medical school at age 18, I had no real understanding of the role I was entering. I had no concept that five years later I would emerge with the responsibility for making decisions about life and death. Deciding who to treat and how, and also who not to treat and why. Discussing diagnoses with people and their families, delivering death sentences. When I was 18 and submitting my polished CV to universities I had no comprehension of the impact this would have on me, the compassion fatigue, the emotional burnout, the sleepless nights, the nightmares. I found over time this didn't get easier, but rather seemed to accumulate into a heavy crushing weight.

The past few years had taken a toll on my mental health. As for many others, the pandemic had been all-consuming and relentless, and although I value my job and the sense of identity it gives me, I increasingly wonder how much longer I can sustain it. As the months went on I found work increasingly draining. I could feel my empathy growing thin and I felt less and less able to give patients the kindness and understanding I knew they deserved. Coming into 2021, I felt like I was sliding steeply downward towards an inescapable cliff edge. As days went by I felt more and more unable to cope. I ran, I saw friends, I ran more, I played the piano, I tried to immerse myself in books, I did yoga, I tried meditation but felt increasingly panicky as the familiar darkness threatened to engulf me. I found myself constantly on the verge of tears and frequently broke down at work. My colleagues were supportive but I felt weak and inadequate. Increasing numbers of staff sickness and isolation meant an already stretched rota became unmanageable and even when I had free time, I was too tired to run and bailed out of routes I had previously done with ease. Finally, inevitably, I reached the breaking point. I caught COVID, and although I wasn't particularly unwell, ten days in isolation by myself pushed me over the edge. I paced my flat, unable to settle to anything. I couldn't concentrate to read or watch films. I barely ate and barely slept, and each day felt like a waking nightmare, filled only with anxiety and unhappiness. On my final day of my isolation, I received a phone call from a friend, informing me that one of our colleagues had committed suicide. Over the next few days I could feel myself unravelling. I went to stay with friends but couldn't find the words to talk about how scared I was. I was constantly consumed by thoughts of her death. I hadn't felt this bad for a number of years, and suddenly all of my thoughts were sucked into my own black hole and I could think of nothing else. I didn't feel safe to be by myself and began to sofa surf between the homes of various friends.

I reach the summit of Red Pike and stop to admire the view. I can see down to the sea in the west and across the expanse of the Lake District. Keswick is nestled out of sight, and looking back across the hills I feel pleased to have run so far. I love to arrive late in my van, rise early, and plot a route on the map, selecting the summits I know I can climb. I take so much pride in feeling that wherever I want to go, my legs will carry me and with a map and compass, I can find my way. The independence and ability to step out into the wild is another reason I love running in the hills.

Thoughts of suicide had been something which had been very real to me in the past. As I had improved and my mood had lifted, this time had felt too intimidating to confront. I had tried to push the memories of that despairing darkness away and hoped it was not a place I would revisit. As I felt myself hurtling downwards over the winter, it was this I was most afraid of. I began to have flashes of this time again. It felt like something that was out of my control, and felt so frightening and overwhelming, and entirely inexpressible. Following the death of my colleague, however, I felt somehow galvanized. I began to speak openly to friends about how I had felt—both in the past and more recently, and found I was not met with horror or repulsion, but warmth and kindness. Others opened up to me about their own feelings and I felt supported in a way I never had before when locked firmly in my own head. Rather than hiding from the thoughts until they overwhelmed me, I began to face them head on and make strategies to keep myself safe.

I climb the broad rocky ridge to gain High Stile. The technical ground once more forces me into the present, as I concentrate on each foot placement, thinking no more than a step ahead, unable to ruminate. I reach the summit and pause. Buttermere lies below me rippling orangey brown, reflecting the increasingly bare autumn trees. To my left the horizon is indistinct, hazing softly into the calm sea. Behind me the ridges and valleys of the lakes look almost infinite; Scafell reaching high beyond Wasdale, appears bare and craggy surrounded by grassier neighbours. It is a view I have come to know well, and the constancy of the familiar hills feels comforting. Surrounded by the majesty of the mountains, my own anxieties are dwarfed into rational proportion. The calm imperialism of the peaks, unwavering by the petty daily irritations of my life, soothes me and helps me find a more comfortable perspective. The dark thoughts which had swirled unstoppable around my mind for weeks finally settled leaving a transparent window of peace and rationality. The knowledge that this calm still can exist brings comfort over the coming weeks. The clouds are not permanent; the darkness contains glimpses of light, however fleeting.

Spring came and the days began to lengthen. I rotated onto a different job and had my weekends free and so began doing regular long hill runs again. One weekend, I suddenly realized that the weight pressing down on me over the preceding months had lifted and I felt I could see clearly again. Over the coming weeks things gradually became easier.

The descent from High Stile is steep and technical, and I concentrate hard, moving slowly downwards through rough boulders and scrambling down narrow ledges, before finally breaking out onto the steep grass and touching down to Buttermere. I'm tiring now and sit at the foot of Robinson to eat. The prospect of another long climb feels daunting, but at this point there is no choice. I secure my pack and climb, slowly now, counting my steps, and resting more often. I feel completely exhausted, but I know I can carry on. I take strength from the fact I know I can push myself and dig down, finding reserves, and pushing forward, far beyond the point of exhaustion. When I return to everyday life, this knowledge that I can keep pushing on beyond my perceived limits transfers. When I feel panicked and unable to cope, I think about the mountains I have climbed despite empty legs, the miles I have pushed through against total exhaustion, and the storms I have endured fighting icy head winds and ploughing on through horizontal rain.

From the summit of Robinson, I can see the remainder of the route. Catbells appears small and achievable, and behind, Keswick nestles along with the promise of tea, cake, and rest. I soar along the grassy ridge feeling elated, confident now I'll complete the round. As I reach the top of Catbells, suddenly the path is busy with people but after a day of relative solitude, this feels friendly rather than oppressive, and I grin at everyone I pass. I begin to push myself as I descend and up my pace through Portinscale, rejoining the road I came out on earlier today. Only nine hours have passed yet I feel renewed and refreshed. I quicken as I enter Keswick, mustering the energy for a short-lived sprint finish to the doors of George Fisher, which I burst through feeling triumphant.

As I sit in my van with a full pint of strong tea, I reflect on the factors which led me here today. Running has carried me through all the difficult times in my life and given me hope even in the darkest times that the sadness will pass. From the strength required to run long distances, I find the strength to cope with difficulties in my day-to-day life. The resilience I have built pursuing long routes year-round in all weather translates into being able to battle on despite the challenges I find in life. I am constantly overwhelmed with gratitude for the people who support me as friends and running partners, and although still fragile, I feel more able to face difficult times ahead. The knowledge that the steadiness and constancy of the mountains awaits me each weekend helps me find perspective in the whirlwind of the week, and being able to escape to the hills gives me resilience to face hard times. I finish my tea and prepare to return to Edinburgh still smiling. This is why I run.

16

Dualisms, Bread and Roses, and Finding Joy

Iona Heath

The Usefulness of Dualisms

I have long been fascinated by the many dualisms and contradictions that permeate medicine (Heath, 1999) and the delivery of healthcare, alongside the notion of a golden mean between contrasting extremes that Aristotle described as the foundation of morality.

The American essayist and philosopher Ralph Waldo Emerson wrote:

> *An inevitable dualism bisects nature, so that each thing is a half, and suggests another thing to make it whole; as, spirit, matter; man, woman; odd, even; subjective, objective; in, out; motion, rest; yea, nay.*

> **(Emerson, 1841)**

And if dualism is fundamental to nature, it must necessarily be fundamental to medicine, especially as new knowledge and understanding tend to accumulate around the borderline within each polarity.

For the purposes of this chapter, my list is completely different, but the point is the same:

- Bread/roses
- Individual ambition/solidarity

DOI: 10.1201/9781003593294-16

- Map/territory
- Word/number
- Transaction/relation

Each polarity creates a potentially destructive tension which can only be resolved through serious dialogue, and so the task for us all becomes to find ways of holding these pairs in a constructive tension.

Getting Things Wrong

Leaving medical school, I thought that all I needed to be a good doctor was a sound grasp of biomedical theory and some capacity for biological reasoning. How wrong could I be?

I remember the particular patient who caused this foundation to crumble under me. We were about the same age—both in our mid-20s—I was a trainee in general practice, and she was a patient who was overwhelmed by anxiety as her life became more and more chaotic and she struggled to cope with a difficult marriage and two young children. I diagnosed her acute thyrotoxicosis, thought I was very clever, started treatment, and assumed that her life would be transformed for the better. Of course, again and by no means for the last time, I was completely wrong. Her physical symptoms of anxiety, the palpitations and disturbed sleep, improved marginally as her thyroid function tests stabilized, but her fundamental predicament was untouched. She remained my patient until I retired so we grew old together: Our children grew up and our parents died. Every time I saw her, I was reminded of my youthful hubris. I remained mostly well while she suffered a succession of chronic autoimmune conditions affecting her skin, her lungs, her joints, and her kidneys and became cushingoid as a result of the corticosteroids she was prescribed by a succession of specialists. Later I learnt about the association of autoimmune conditions with adverse child experiences, and this made some sense of her situation (Kirkengen, 2010).

Slowly and sometimes painfully, I learnt that biomedical knowledge is essential but by no means sufficient for the practice of medicine. I learnt about the overwhelming power of biography to damage biology irreversibly, and I came to understand the power of the intersubjective relationship between two unique individuals, one a doctor and the other a patient. I discovered that the careful nurturing of this relationship through the paying of real attention has the capacity to help people to feel better about themselves and more confident in their ability to cope even in situations where biomedicine has very little to offer. And this became the story of my relationship with this particular patient and, I hope, many others over half a lifetime. We liked each other and we forgave each other our inadequacies, and it helped us both.

Bread/Roses

Bread is what makes life possible, and roses are what makes life worth living.

In the middle of March 2024, I went to see an exhibition at the Royal Academy of Art in London titled *Entangled Pasts, 1768–Now: Art, Colonialism and Change*. I was thinking about the challenge of writing this chapter and, perhaps because of this, I was most struck by Zanzibar-born British artist Lubaina Himid's extraordinary installation called "Naming the Money" and originally created in 2004.

The work filled a whole large room and was made up of 100 brightly painted, life-size, cut-out figures, each representing the story of an individual slave. Pasted on the back of each cutout was a small balance sheet. All the sums are recorded as $0.00, underlining the harsh reality of slavery, but under "Item description," we seem to hear the voice of the particular slave. A dog trainer says:

My name is Adeban
They call me Sam
I used to jump through waves.
Now I teach dogs to guard
But I have their love.

A painter says:

My name is Kwaboaso
They call me Polly
I painted patterns on my house
Now I keep their woodwork nice
But I have the shadows.

Each slave has had their past, and even their name, obliterated, yet despite the horror of their situation, each finds some comfort, even some joy, in the last line of their statement.

I thought to myself that each of these last lines are examples of what I am calling roses, illustrating the powerful human need to find some joy in life, however grim the circumstances. And when I look back, I think that both my patient and I found roses as well as bread as our relationship unfolded.

Bread and roses emerged as a political slogan in the United States around 1910 and was used by women campaigning for votes for women. In September 1911, a New York daily magazine explained the use of the slogan in the growing campaign for women's suffrage:

> *Her vote will go toward helping forward the time when life's Bread, which is home, shelter and security, and the Roses of life—music, education, nature and books— shall be the heritage of every child that is born in the country in the government of which she has a voice.*
>
> **(Evening World, 1911)**

The then 28-year-old American poet James Oppenheim was inspired to turn the slogan into a poem that was first published in December 1911.

It has since become a well-known protest song which ends with the lines:

> *Small art and love and beauty*
> *Their drudging spirits knew*
> *Yes, it is bread we fight for*
> *But we fight for roses too.*
>
> **(Oppenheim, 1911)**

In her recent book (Solnit, 2021), *Orwell's Roses*, the American essayist Rebecca Solnit wrote an entire section exploring the history and implications of the slogan. She was inspired to write the book when she discovered that George Orwell had not only written the bleakest and most powerful portrayals of the totalitarian regimes of the twentieth century but had also planted rose bushes, costing sixpence each from Woolworths. She writes:

> *Bread fed the body, roses fed something subtler: not just hearts, but imaginations, psyches, senses, identities. It was a pretty slogan but a fierce argument that more than survival and bodily well-being were needed and were being demanded as a right. It was equally an argument against the idea that everything that human beings need can be reduced to quantifiable, tangible goods and conditions. Roses in these declarations stood for the way that human beings are complex, desires are irreducible, that what sustains us is often subtle and elusive.*

When my friend Peruvian American physician Victor Montori suggested that I read this book, he could see immediately its relevance to the current state of healthcare in his country and in mine. Together, we wrote:

> *"Bread and roses" are what the humans involved in care—the patient and the clinician—want from healthcare. Bread is sustenance and therefore life; roses are courage and hope, curiosity and joy, and all that makes a life worth living. Bread is biology; roses are biography. Bread is transactional and technocratic; roses are relational. Bread is science; roses are care, kindness and love.*
>
> **(Heath & Montori, 2023)**

This understanding of the politics of bread and roses seems entirely relevant not only to the state of much healthcare today but to the predicament of doctors and patients within it, because when there are no roses but only bread, the relational gives way to the transactional and all manner of distress is treated with pharmaceuticals and other medical technologies, and clinicians begin to suffer moral injury.

A human being is both a subject and an object—and that includes all patients and all doctors. Bread and roses are needed by everyone. As so many of the previous chapters have shown, both are essential—one alone is never enough, and each of us has to find the right balance between them in order to achieve not only life, but a life worth living. And it seems to me that, within too much healthcare, there has been a diminishing supply of roses for both patients and doctors over recent years, maligned in Solnit's words as:

> Trivial, irrelevant, indulgent, pointless, distracted, or any of those other pejoratives with which the quantifiable beats down the unquantifiable.

How has this been allowed to happen, when it is the roses that help to build trusting therapeutic relationships and to mitigate suffering? Perhaps because healthcare with universal coverage can only flourish within a politics of solidarity.

Individual Ambition/Solidarity: The Terrible Legacy of Neoliberal Economics

Last year, Abby Innes, associate professor in political economy at the London School of Economics, published a book with the rather shocking title *Late Soviet Britain* (Innes, 2023). I found it quite remarkably helpful in making so much more sense of what happened to the UK National Health Service (NHS) during my 35-year career as a general practitioner in Kentish Town in London. Of course, I knew that the rot set in with Margaret Thatcher, and I listened to Julian Le Grand, Tony Blair's favourite health economist, saying that I was never a knight but always a knave, never altruistic, always self-interested (Le Grand, 2003), but I had never clocked the almost unbelievable stupidity of the underlying neoliberal economics—it just felt as if we were all having the rug pulled out from under us more and more with every passing year.

Innes draws a convincing parallel between the Soviet utopia of Leninist central planning after the 1917 revolution and the neoliberal utopia promulgated by the Chicago School of Economics in the 1970s. Both relied on conceptions of the political economy as a perfect mechanism, ruled by predetermined laws of economic behaviour that were used to promote pure systems of economic coordination be that by the state or the market. Both relied on magical thinking, and she points out one of the many ironies:

> Most remarkably of all, the neoliberal project would take hold through the 1970s, just as the Soviet planning system was demonstrating beyond a shadow of a doubt that governance systems based on closed-system reasoning were a recipe for quite staggering political and economic dysfunction.

In the first paragraph of her book, she writes:

The shattering of the British state over the last forty years was driven by the idea that markets are always more efficient than the state: the private sector morally and functionally superior to the public sector.

And I immediately see the truth of this through the lens of the NHS.

On the next page she writes:

When it comes to the mechanics of government, both systems justify a near identical methodology of quantification, forecasting, target setting and output-planning.

and

Since the world in practice is dynamic and synergistic, . . . it follows that the state's increasing reliance on methods that presume rational calculation within an unvarying underlying universal order can only lead to a continuous misfit between governmental theory and reality. These techniques will tend to fail around any task characterised by uncertainty, intricacy, interdependence and evolution.

And to the extent that these are precisely the characteristics of healthcare, the whole history of the last 40 years of the NHS and many other healthcare systems around the world takes on a horrifying clarity.

Neoliberal Economics Have Made Doctors into Little More Than Drug-Pushers

The bizarre foundational idea of neoliberal economics is the notion of perfect competition which was supposed to function magically for the benefit of all by exploiting the virtues of the market and rejecting the so-called pathologies of cooperation. This belief in markets as a moral good has worked, perversely, to legitimize greed and the unfettered pursuit of profit, and the whole enterprise has worked for the massive benefit of the very few while causing untold harm to the very many.

Over the past 40 years, freed by the delusions of neoliberalism, the pharmaceutical and medical technology industries have pursued profit with commitment, enthusiasm, and absolutely staggering success. Any idea of working for the benefit of all has long been lost, and it seems astonishing to remember the 1955 interview in which Jonas Salk was asked who owned the patent for the inactivated polio vaccine that he had developed. He replied:

Well, the people, I would say. There is no patent. Could you patent the sun?

Today, the pharmaceutical industry is one of the most profitable in the world, and it has energetically adopted the neoliberal hallmarks of financialization and tax evasion. An investigation of the world's 27 largest pharmaceutical companies (Fernandez & Klinge, 2020) shows that, over the last 20 years, more money was invested in financial activities than in medicine production and research. In total, US$1540 billion was paid to shareholders between 2000 and 2018. At the ten largest pharmaceutical companies, the overall distribution of funds to shareholders was 142% higher than the amount spent on research and development in a given year. Again, the few are doing very well! And, on top of this, around 75% of the pharmaceutical industry's income is reported offshore for tax purposes. Even compared to other multinationals, the profit shifting and the lack of concern for social welfare of pharmaceutical companies are extreme.

Yet even more relevant to those struggling within medicine is the legacy of the brilliance with which the medical–industrial complex has managed to restructure healthcare in its own interests. There have been three principal methods in play: First, persuading clinicians to treat risk of disease as a disease in itself in the name of prevention; second, persuading policymakers to track, incentivize, and control healthcare activity; and finally, funding special interest and guideline groups to equate quality standards with levels of testing and/or prescribing. These tactics have been devastatingly successful, producing an avalanche of polypharmacy, with little evidence of benefit to individual patients, and leaving an ever-increasing number of doctors feeling that they are doing little more than pushing drugs. In the process, doctors and other clinicians have allowed the wisdom of centuries in relation to care, caution and minimizing harm to be almost totally eroded.

In her book *Held*, which was short-listed for the 2024 Booker Prize, the magnificent Canadian poet and novelist Anne Michaels warns us all about . . .

> *The avarice of science, its conflation of knowledge and control.*
>
> **(Michaels, 2023)**

A conflation that troubles so many clinicians.

Standing on the Shoulders of Giants

We all rely on the shoulders of particular giants in our struggle to understand and find meaning in our experience, and, clearly, I am already standing on the shoulders of Rebecca Solnit and Abby Innes, with more to come. In relation to my experience of general practice, one of the most important of my giants has been Ian McWhinney, who left general practice in England to become the inaugural chair of family medicine at the University of Western Ontario in 1968. I first heard him speak when he gave the 1996 William Pickles Lecture for the UK Royal College of GPs (McWhinney, 1996), and I knew immediately that his strikingly narrow shoulders would prove invaluable to me and to those whom, in my turn, I sought to teach. In the lecture he referred to many of his own intellectual inspirations, and he included the Polish American philosopher and scientist Alfred Korzybski.

Map/Territory

In 1933, Korzybski wrote:

> *A map is not the territory it represents, but, if correct, it has a similar structure to the territory, which accounts for its usefulness.*
>
> **(Korzybski, 1933)**

In 1996, McWhinney developed this idea, saying:

> *We cannot experience the beauty or the terror of a landscape by reading the map. . . . If we are to be healers as well as technicians, we have at some point to set aside our maps and walk hand-in-hand with our patients through the territory.*

As witnessed in the previous chapters, many of the problems within contemporary medicine follow from our increasing obsession with the seductive but deceptive certainties of our theoretical map and our growing neglect of the territory of illness and suffering. So much current research involves adding more and more detail to the map, and the ever-exploding map takes ever more attention in teaching. There is an urgent need to redress the balance and attempt to broaden our wisdom and understanding in relation to the realities of the particular suffering in the individual lives of our patients.

The American physician Eric Cassell wrote:

We all recognize certain injuries that almost invariably cause suffering: the death or suffering of loved ones, powerlessness, helplessness, hopelessness, torture, the loss of a life's work, deep betrayal, physical agony, isolation, homelessness, memory failure, and unremitting fear. Each touches features common to us all, yet each contains features that must be defined in terms of a specific person at a specific time.

(Cassell, 1991)

Every working day, doctors listen to people who tell stories of suffering mediated by each one of these causes, and we know the power of suffering to undermine both joy and hope, leaving a life in tatters. Clinicians also suffer, perhaps most of all at the hands of fear and betrayal. The fear of making a mistake and harming a patient haunts us throughout our careers. Betrayal is more difficult to recognize, but we feel it whenever our aspirations to be good doctors are actively undermined by the systems within which we work.

A disconnect between the map and the territory, similar to that experienced by patients, is also present in the working lives of clinicians, where the artificial clarity of the delivery models imposed by policymakers feels a far cry from the chaos and ambiguity of daily practice. This disconnect is scarcely ever acknowledged in political rhetoric, which only serves to increase the distress and suffering of clinicians.

Abby Innes recognizes this situation as a feature of neoliberalism which:

introduces a systematic analytical bias that leads governments to increasingly mistake the closed-system map for the open-system terrain over which they govern.

And just how often have we seen this bias at play in those policy documents that seem so out of touch with the reality of working lives in medicine?

Some of this complete lack of understanding of the territory of healthcare is revealed in a recent ethnographic study of "hidden work" in general practice, work which is integral to direct patient care but not patient-facing and which takes up almost 30% of GP time (Barnard et al., 2024). It includes, among much else, interpreting test results, crafting referrals, and accepting interruptions from clinical colleagues.

The study highlighted the difficulties that GPs confront in this hidden, unrecognized, and unremunerated work, and, as Peter Dorward describes when checking test results in Chapter 3.3, it is hedged in by ambiguity and clinical uncertainty.

The irreducible uncertainty inherent in GPs' work extends to hidden care work just as it characterises direct patient care. Direct and hidden care work often fold into each other in practices such as diagnostic decision-making which require GPs to interpret and synthesise fragments of information relating to unique individuals. Good practice in primary care requires GPs to switch between speed-work and deliberative-work.

(Barnard et al., 2024)

When working conditions make it impossible to switch in this way, GPs suffer distress and fear, making mistakes because they remain aware that they are simply skating over the surface of what needs to be done.

Other research by the same team investigated the separation between the map and the territory in the context of medication reviews for older people subjected to polypharmacy (Pocknell et al., 2024). In this situation, the map mandates a bureaucratic procedure aimed at revisiting the need for medication and reducing the number and amount of medication prescribed. In stark contrast, the territory presents the mostly unarticulated fears of ageing, disease, and death within a context of years of being told that the prescribed drugs were essential to treat or reduce the risk of serious disease and, by implication, death.

Moral Injury

In his book 2013 book on *The Nature of Healing*, Eric Cassell writes:

The care of patients is a moral undertaking or perhaps a moral-technical one. That is because what is done must be in the best interests of the patients—what is good and right for patients—as they know them. Good and right are words in the moral world, they are not technical issues even though technical knowledge may be required for their achievement.

(Cassell, 2013)

Yet within the neoliberal political context, the definition of morality, like so much else, has been hollowed out and diminished. Abby Innes writes:

The new moral philosophy of utilitarianism was that we should understand what was morally right or wrong by what caused us pleasure as opposed to pain. An act was morally virtuous if it produced a net gain in pleasure. Moral decision-making could thus be reduced to a cost-benefit analysis.

(Innes, 2023)

Yet despite this miserable context, most physicians continue to cling to Cassell's view within a vocational ethos of public service. The result is widespread demoralization and pervasive moral injury, so clearly understood by Innes:

When institutional architectures are misconceived but enforced as "scientific" doctrine, then rational people are incentivised to do damaging things, and conscientious people are forced to spend huge additional effort to limit the harm inflicted by the systems within which they work.

(Innes, 2023)

Science depends on its grounding in reality, and theory and practice need to rotate to achieve scientific progress. Any constraints on the representation and interpretation of how theory plays out in practice curtails the scope for adaptive learning and correction, following trial, error, and review, which together constitute the scientific method. The whole enterprise is threatened when the gap between the map and the territory becomes too great and when there is less and less room for imagination, creativity, experience, and wise judgement.

Words/Numbers

Numbers have a beauty and purity that are very seductive and give an impression of solidity and certainty. Words, on the other hand, are infinitely malleable and adaptable to circumstance. We have begun to define disease by means of number, and this has separated the map from the territory to an even greater extent.

This supremacy of number is yet another legacy of contemporary neoliberalism which depends on quantification and using numbers to atomize society and reduce patients, doctors, consultations, treatments, and everything else you can think of into interacting units within a closed economic system, completely out of touch with the realities of sickness and healthcare.

Transactional/Relational

In view of the powerful interactions between biology and biography within every story of illness or disease, there has to be a balance in clinical practice between the transactional bread and the relational roses if medical care is to be effective.

This transactional/relational balance was in place when I started out but had been severely damaged by the time I stopped, as bureaucratic imperatives and technological change allowed the transactional to displace the relational and number to displace words.

Physicians must become enchanted by the wonders of those persons who are patients, rather than bewitched by the marvels of science.

(Fuks et al., 2012)

The transactional nature of biomedical science has nothing to offer suffering, and only our relational skills can help.

As James Baldwin wrote in his 1964 book with the photographer Richard Avedon:

I have always felt that a human being could only be saved by another human being. I am aware that we do not save each other very often. But I am also aware that we save each other some of the time.

(Avedon & Baldwin, 1964)

It is a disturbing irony that the importance of relational care, which is so dependent on the exchange of words and already so self-evident to those in clinical practice, has only begun to be accepted, to a still very limited extent, by politicians and policymakers since its validation by quantitative research.

This was achieved by a registry-based observational study conducted in Norway which provided strong evidence that continuity of care by a regular general practitioner is associated with reduced need for out-of-hours services and acute hospital admission and decreased mortality in a dose-dependent way. If the GP–patient relationship has lasted >15 years, the probability of these occurrences is reduced by 25–30% (Sandvik et al., 2022).

These are stunning findings, making continuing relational care more effective than all the drugs prescribed for asymptomatic people in the name of prevention.

The Way Forward

How are we to reassert the importance of roses alongside the essential bread of medicine and rediscover the joy in our work? I have tried to suggest that we need to learn from a multitude of different disciplines outside medicine including art, music, literature, philosophy, ethnography, and even economics.

James Baldwin explained the essential nature of art in this way:

> *A society must assume that it is stable, but the artist must know, and he must let us know, that there is nothing stable under heaven. One cannot possibly build a school, teach a child, or drive a car without taking some things for granted. The artist cannot and must not take anything for granted, but must drive to the heart of every answer and expose the question the answer hides.*
>
> **(Baldwin, 1962)**

If the answer was neoliberal economics, I dread to imagine the question because I fear it was how to make money for the few at the expense of the many. Baldwin underlines the extent to which doctors need help from artists in order to challenge our more superficial understandings of the nature of power, our society, and the predicament of our patients.

Research needs to be rebalanced so that the territory is scrutinized as much as, if not more so than, the map. As Deborah Swinglehurst has shown, careful, painstaking ethnographic studies can reveal aspects of the territory that are not really seen even by those struggling to survive there, both as patients and professionals.

In this book, we have tried to take every opportunity to confront the purveyors of the map with stories from the territory. Only by insisting on researching the territory and reporting back our experience of it, again both as patients and professionals, can we have any hope of closing the gap between it and the map or of resisting the pernicious effects of neoliberal economic nonsense.

We need to nurture the doubt and uncertainty that are anathema to the self-righteous utopian thinking of neoliberalism, and, oddly, there is joy and freedom to be found in doubt and uncertainty. Rebecca Solnit reminds us that there is also hope:

> *Hope locates itself in the premises that we don't know what will happen and that in the spaciousness of uncertainty is room to act. When you recognize uncertainty, you recognize that you may be able to influence the outcomes—you alone or you in concert with a few dozen or several million others. Hope is an embrace of the unknown and the unknowable, an alternative to the certainty of both optimists and pessimists.*
>
> **(Solnit, 2016)**

We need to identify, record, research, and teach all those elements of practice that bring joy into the consultation, including perhaps those moments when curiosity leads to an almost blinding flash of insight into the patient's predicament but also those spent listening to stories of infinite and fascinating variety, which enable us to see the other in a completely different light; discovering the young person still lurking within the old and frail survivor in front of us; rediscovering the fascination and privilege of home visits; finding the courage to prevent harm by resisting the seductions of over-testing, overdiagnosis, and overtreatment; feeling the satisfaction of knowing that a procedure was undertaken skilfully or that a correct diagnosis was made, the rare but simple sensation of a job well done; and much, much more.

And in all these ways:

Yes, it is bread we fight for

But we fight for roses too.

References

Avedon, R., & Baldwin, J. (1964). *Nothing personal.* Atheneum.

Baldwin, J. (1985). The creative process. In J. Baldwin (Ed.), *The price of the ticket: Collected nonfiction 1948–1985.* St Martin's Press. (Original work published 1962)

Barnard, R., Spooner, S., Hubmann, M., Checkland, K., Campbell, J., & Swinglehurst, D. (2024). The hidden work of general practitioners: An ethnography. *Social Science & Medicine, 350,* 116922.

Cassell, E. (1991). *The nature of suffering and the goals of medicine.* Oxford University Press.

Cassell, E. (2013). *The nature of healing: The modern practice of medicine.* Oxford Univeristy Press.

Emerson, R. W. (1841). *Essays* (1st series, vol. 1, 1st ed., T. Carlyle, Ed.).

Fernandez, R., & Klinge, T. J. (2020). *Private gains we can ill afford: The financialisation of big pharma.* www.somo.nl

Fuks, A., Brawer, J., & Boudreau, J. D. (2012). The foundation of physicianship. *Perspectives in Biology and Medicine, 55*(1), 114–126.

Heath, I. (1999). 'Uncertain clarity': Contradiction, meaning, and hope. *British Journal of General Practice, 49,* 651–657.

Heath, I., & Montori, V. M. (2023). Responding to the crisis of care. *BMJ, 380,* 464. https://doi.org/10.1136/bmj.p464

Innes, A. (2023). *Late soviet Britain.* Cambridge University Press.

Kirkengen, A. L. (2010). *The lived experience of violation: How abused children become unhealthy adults.* Zeta Books.

Korzybski, A. (1933). *Science and Sanity: An introduction to non-Aristotelian systems and general semantics.* Institute of General Semantics.

Le Grand, J. (2003). *Motivation, agency, and public policy: Of knights and knaves, pawns and queens.* Oxford University Press.

McWhinney, I. R. (1996). The importance of being different. *British Journal of General Practice, 46,* 433–436.

Michaels, A. (2023). *Held.* Bloomsbury Publishing.

Pocknell, S., Fudge, N., Collins, S., Roberts, C., & Swinglehurst, D. (2024). 'Troubling' medication reviews in the context of polypharmacy and ageing: A linguistic ethnography. *Social Science & Medicine, 352,* 117025. https://doi.org/10.1016/j.socscimed.2024.117025

Sandvik, H., Hetlevik, Ø., Blinkenberg, J., & Hunskaar, S. (2022). Continuity in general practice as predictor of mortality, acute hospitalisation, and use of out-of-hours care: A registry-based observational study in Norway. *British Journal of General Practice, 72*(715), e84–e90.

Solnit, R. (2016). *Hope in the dark: Untold histories, wild possibilities.* Haymarket Books.

Solnit, R. (2021). *Orwell's roses.* Granta Books.

17

The Planning of Magic

Edvin Schei and Peter Dorward

Introduction

The form of this chapter is a conversation—a dialogue that takes place during a walk up a rugged green mountain in Scotland. Up, then down again. As we climbed rocky trails and splashed through murky swamps, we sought through years of experience, trying to identify and formulate rules of thumb that might help others plan and prepare professional gatherings, where the goal was to have meetings of minds—meetings of equals, irrespective of hierarchy—which resulted in change—and not mere displays of cleverness, or expertise, or power.

After the walk, we recorded our thoughts. We summed things up over a cup of tea, a slice of cake, in the garden of a falling-down country house in Perthshire, Scotland.

That was our methodology.

It was early autumn. The recording of our talking is alive with birdsong. You can hear a wood pigeon. A blackbird in the alto range. A song-thrush, its great diversity of calls and rhythms, no two groups of calls the same. And two characters analysing the medico-philosophical conferences that they were both involved in organizing during the previous 18 months, first in Rosendal in the west of Norway, then in Roshven in the west of Scotland. Call it the RosRos symposia.

The two events gathered a diverse group of about 14 doctors from various countries, some young, some old, to wrestle with questions of what

DOI: 10.1201/9781003593294-17

constitutes the core, the best values and practices in healing and medicine. What, if anything, is "The Right Stuff of Medicine," and how can we sustain and protect that stuff in a world and time where it seems threatened? The symposia were meticulously planned to promote an environment fertile with ideas, trust, and creativity. It worked well, twice. We think we know why it worked, we think we could repeat it, and we think others can do likewise.

The planning took time and a great deal of commitment. We, an organizing group of five enthusiastic physicians, challenged ourselves to clarify our purposes and identify the weaknesses in our own proposals, allowing for disagreements, even for conflict, to fertilize our discussions and expand our collective thinking.

People, when they're vulnerable, get defensive. People can be easily bored. Moods that block participation and creativity. We needed to be prepared for that. And we, the organizers, needed a willingness to accept that, although planning is crucial, elaborate plans are no guarantee of success. *The best-laid schemes o' mice an' men gang aft agley.* There has to be jeopardy, and it must be real. Like any other handicraft, clinical medicine—for example, the running of a conference—is characterized by risk; guesses, intuitions, improvisations, conflicts, reconciliations. Lose the risk, and you lose the creativity, the stretching of minds, the learning and innovation that were the point of it all. The most important outcome of prolonged planning may not be the draft program, but the leaders' mental preparedness and trust in each other. Both are crucial for dealing with the unpredictable problems that will come.

The purpose of the RosRos symposia was to have a group of young and old physicians from different countries think honestly and openly together about what "The Right Stuff of Medicine" might be. Apparently, thinking is the easy bit. We cannot stop even if we want to. But to do it honestly— with courage, humility—about personally disturbing questions, with our vulnerable, fallible, fumbling stupidities always at play—that is not so easy. We're proud folk, all of us. We become defensive, wordy, strategic. We can seek to impress and control, to be validated, admired. Changed? Perhaps not so much. That's really hard.

Twice then, in 2022 and 2023, we, our group, got together and wrestled with those philosophical questions, and with our own emotions, blind spots, defences. We came up with some tentative answers, some of which have found their way into this book. But essential though these questions and answers might have been, they weren't the whole point. Our ambitions were greater, and more practical.

We think (and we're not the first) that although "good and right answers"—also known as knowledge—are crucial, they have little value if not embodied in practice. "Wisdom" has no virtue unless it's also doing. How often as students, or doctors, have we believed that we "know" what we ought to do, or feel, or be, yet can't act on this knowledge?

Burnout, cynicism, and misery are legion in medicine, and they have many causes (see Chapter 12). We believe these problems originate, at least in part, from the dissociation of the technical practice of medicine, from its moral and emotional value—the value of difficult things like care. The best manner by which that value might be known is through its continuous regeneration, in caring and challenging interactions of committed, open, vulnerable minds. People need to *feel* and be moved to recognize value and be tempted to act on it (see Chapter 10). Simply telling folk what to do never, ever works. But trusting interaction between participants at a seminar doesn't happen just by magic serendipity—the preconditions for magic must be crafted. Ideally, all doctors should be able to craft some magic and know how to heal. These were among our ambitions for the conferences.

Magic did happen. There were music and singing, there was swimming in the sea, which was warm still, clear, deep, blue, and kind to us. The sun shone, the food was good. There were irritations too, bickering, people feeling left out, latent conflicts, moments of real jeopardy and suffering. There were misgivings, and there were blunders and wrong steps. But trust grows if the soil is fertile, if mistakes are admitted and people taken seriously. Some delegates left emboldened. Many inspired. A few felt transformed. Newly strong—with knowledge, skills, new perspectives. How much easier it felt to face the hard faceless present, after such a hard-won meeting of minds! Yet how un-measurable are these benefits! And how intangible those many, shifting choices and decisions, funnelled through volatile human dynamics, that contribute to success or failure. If it went well, as it did, can we claim it was more than pure luck? Which aspects of the planning were really important? And, if we succeeded, can such a success be translated to other settings where clinicians and educators need to think well and act wisely?

Cast of Characters

Edvin, a GP and professor of medicine from Bergen (who had a hunch that things would work out well).

Peter, a GP and author from Edinburgh (who was filled with crippling doubts about the whole enterprise but got through it).

A wise old woman, eating a banana.

Part 1: Joy

We walk past the grounds of a stately mansion house, backed onto the shores of a loch. The woman of the house, eccentric, aristocratic, is said to keep a domesticated owl in her kitchen. At night it swoops from the rafters to terrorize the mice that gather to feast on the crumbs on her unswept floor.

We pass a gravestone, marking the site where a group of Macdonald highlanders were slaughtered by ancestors of the owners of the estate, the Clan Stewart of Appin, for the crime of stealing cattle. The stone stands obscured by undergrowth; the writing chiselled on its surface almost worn flat. In a few years, all memory of these bloody events will be lost.

Peter: So . . . where should we start? I felt completely transformed by the whole RosRos experience, and I know others did too. We're thinking that the better we understand how it happened, the better, both for ourselves and for future organizers of comparable events. Edvin, you've organized similarly intense symposia several times before. Medical philosophy and powerful change is your thing. What are your thoughts? How does it get done?

Edvin is experiencing a moment of gratitude for finding himself in another adventure. About to embark on a long day of walking and talking with this thoughtful Scottish doctor, a far reach from those narrow Norwegian fjords and those narrow, technical, academic ideas of what it means to be, to become, a healer.

Edvin: I think we underestimate the importance of people's feelings in learning situations, as well as in healing. We put all the emphasis on the cognitive content—is the knowledge presented by teachers and lecturers—or physicians—correct and relevant, engaging and clear? I agree that the content and the style of presentation are important. But it just isn't enough. I think that deserves to be talked about today.

Peter: Unpack that. What do you mean by "not enough?"

Edvin: Well, our conferences needed high-quality content—the deep knowledge of highly skilled senior colleagues, the stories from the trenches that were told by the youngest doctors, and the powerful ideas and theories of human behaviour that were discussed. However, the crucial thing for participants' minds and hearts to truly open were the moods, the feelings, the power that can emerge from the dynamics between people. Only if they were emotionally touched would they open up to change—believe in their own critical judgement, be transformed by ideas, grow stronger. In addition to content, we needed to provide, somehow, a bedrock of psychological safety, a felt freedom to be honest, spontaneous, to think on the spot, say strange and unfinished things, without losing face. I would like to talk with you about *how* that was achieved and how we think it can be achieved in other places, in different contexts.

Peter: I agree. Those dynamics between the participants and the emotional states that you talk about, they were generated and protected by the framework of activities and rest that we had set up, the preparations we had involved everybody in, and how we used our position as leaders to guide all of us through the days. But things went wrong too. Do you remember how tired everybody was on that first day? How hunger, over-planning, too many hours on the road caused irritation and threatened to damage everything? I had to leave the meeting that first night. Do you remember? I thought that I'd let you all down, screwed everything up. I went for a swim with Lizzie. That was healing. But definitely not in the plan! But then there was the beauty of the fjord, the layout of the buildings, the quality of the meals, the singing and poetry in the evenings. And the weather, of course! What did we do to get a whole week of sun on the west coast of Scotland? Truly a brilliant achievement!

Edvin: That's a business secret, not to be divulged.

As the two figures ascend the green hill, there is a gentle incline, just enough to make you a little breathless. The mountain ahead makes a satisfying pyramid, the summit lost in the last of the morning's mist. It provokes in Edvin a recollection of a hike he took last autumn from his cabin in the hills above Oster Fjord with his son and then a secondary recollection: Of the patch of cloudberries that they had found there, nested in the lichen, how bitter and sweet they were on the tongue.

Peter: OK, we won't tell. But seriously, how can we convey the ambitions we had, what we wanted to avoid, and how we consciously attempted to make these events different, more rewarding and impactful, than most conferences? We agree that the emotional aspect is central to human thinking and learning—but why, and how? That's clearly not the message that we got during our medical education.

Edvin: Well, as doctors we supposedly know a lot about people, but we also share plenty of professional blind spots. Understanding the role of emotions is one of them. Human beings are emotional all the time; that's an aspect of our existential anatomy (Rudebeck, 2001). We are constantly in some kind of mood, we always react—with emotions of attraction or repulsion, interest or boredom, anger, worry or joy—to everything that happens to us. Emotions are shortcut cognitions, they show us the world in a flash, rightly or wrongly perceived, and they steer our reactions (Kahneman, 2011). But medical education tends to shy away from emotion, treat emotion in students and physicians as a taboo, a sign of weakness. So medical teachers and students make it a habit to keep a stiff upper lip and control themselves. Some scholars contend that doctors are contaminated with "alexithymia" during their formation (Shapiro, 2011). That's to say, unable to understand and use emotional signals in human communication. Not a very helpful habit, to put it mildly, if your job is to help people in deep crises. Nor if you want to inspire interest, reflection, and increased wisdom in people, which is what medical education and academic conferences are ostensibly about.

Peter: Yeah. The problem's deeply built in. That fear of shame and weakness, of feeling too much, getting caught out. I was like that for years. I get the occasional relapse. You think there's something wrong with you. You keep having these intense, inconvenient *emotions*. So you suppress it, or you're just unhappy and alone while everybody else seems to be doing fine. It's systemic, and it's "the wrong stuff of medicine." So let's talk about how we used this "emotional knowledge" in our quest for The Right Stuff to happen in the RosRos seminars!

Edvin: Let's start with joy. I have a friend whose motto is "it's more fun to have fun than not to have fun." I am equally childish; I want learning to be joyful, even when it's about very serious and even painful topics. So we aimed for joy—first by a fjord in Rosendal and then by a fjord in the north-west of Scotland. Now we are trying to tell the story about how that was done— how a safe place was created where we, being very serious and very vulnerable people, could for a moment lose our stiffness and be playful again, while earnestly struggling to understand the complexity of our professional experiences better. We sought joy, not to entertain or distract ourselves, but as a necessary state of mind for exploring together that which seems confusing, bewildering, and uncertain, in search of better insights and greater wisdom. Joyful thinking entails motivation, patience, stamina, collaboration, support, which of course elicit feelings of joy—it's a self-perpetuating spiral, if it succeeds. Any toddler engaged in play can show us that. As I think about it and recall what it felt like to be in that state, I get this sense of energy and power. I wouldn't be surprised if participating in such processes make people *better* at everything they do.

Peter: Better. At everything you do. That's a whopper of a big claim.

Edvin: Big claim, yes, and I don't know where it came from, I just heard myself say it. Probably a crazy claim. Let's mull over it, we have the whole day ahead of us.

They walk in silence for a bit, catching their breath, finding their stride. Each thinking, alone, about emotional knowledge. Knowing, through joy? Pleasure, a tool for learning? And how would the world look if that could be made true?

A brief pause, as they look at the scenery below them.

Peter: I don't want to spoil the mood, but I think we need something a bit tangible. You've arranged similar things for more than 20 years. If you think through those events, what would you say is the common red thread? Take your time, give me some bullet points.

Delivers each point every few paces, interspersed by moments of rest, the drinking in of air, the increasingly glorious autumn colour:

Edvin: Have an organizing group, people with energy—intellectual enthusiasm and sense of adventure, people who like and trust each other. That's the culture for the sourdough of relational dynamics that you want to create.

Start planning a year or more in advance.

Agree on a theme that is exciting.

Find a venue that is secluded, so that the participants will spend time together, have meals together, sleep in the same place.

Decide on the length of the symposium. I recommend three to four days, plus travel time. It takes time for people to get through the initial ice breaking, then become involved in thinking about the theme, then start to share and elaborate their own experiences, and then converge in the production of results: Reflections, discussions, connections, insights.

Find a funding source. Individuals, institutions, grants.

Invite participants and presenters. Be aware that the wording of invitations by email or otherwise is a pivotal stage.

Peter: I remember that invitation process. The care that we took in the drafting and re-drafting, the tone, that balance of giving and withholding of information, the cultivating of a sense of mystery, playfulness, inspiration, challenge, seriousness, excitement. These email invitations were works of art in themselves. I guess they're always going to be different— adapted for the purpose of the event and the community that's being built.

Edvin: The magic must be made. And then it must be made again. It's real work, it can take an hour, or a week, to craft that first sentence, the one that sparks your energy and makes it easy to write a paragraph.

Peter: No two times the same.

Edvin: I guess.

Peter: A thing I *do* remember, and I think that it needs to be stated, was the special, extraordinary status of these meetings of minds and of bodies. We were all of us standing outside of our ordinary lives. Unfamiliar places, somewhat unfamiliar people, that feeling of being separate from the world, that enabled transformation. There was no one dropping in or out, no one on devices, no Zooming, everyone was present. That was a precondition for success.

Edvin: And an outcome of all that planning.

Peter: A desired, but by no means inevitable, outcome.

Edvin: And the transitions—those points of potential friction, as the group formed, and as it broke apart again.

Peter: Actually—it wasn't easy. Again, I remember that first night, the realization that we had potential conflict. I thought that there was a risk that people were going to get really angry. We were asking too much. They were tired, and we hadn't really allowed for that.

Did we get that right though? Really?

Edvin: I think we made some dangerous mistakes in the beginning. We were worried and tired. Stubbornly and anxiously we followed plans instead of asking the participants for help, as we could and should have done. I will do it differently another time. But there will be other mistakes, as long as I live. It's unavoidable, predictable, yet totally embarrassing when it happens—it's never "the right mistake." Knowing that, and facing it, means to be willing to show people respect by meeting their eyes, listen, say that you're sorry and mean it, and change plans if need be. It's humbling, quite uncomfortable, and necessary. We did that. And as often happens, relationships were more robust, more trusting, after we had survived that conflict.

Now we are in mixed woodland, a river tumbles to our left. The gradient steepens, the path somewhat winding. The conversation is beginning to be more free-flowing.

Peter: You can't think clearly about a thing unless you have the words or language to express the thought. We doctors have a cognitive repertoire that allows fluency in certain areas, but makes us stumbling and hesitant in others. One of the ends of this whole thing was to allow for access to different, unfamiliar kinds of thinking.

Edvin, thinking, *but do I agree? What am I agreeing to? Language? What does that even mean? But let it go. For now.*

Edvin: As medical students or physicians we might have our wordless suspicions that something is wrong, something about how we're formed as doctors—but we're fearful, or powerless, or we lack confidence to follow through on these fears. The cognitive dissonance makes us powerless to act—we become avoidant of the pain that such insight can create.

Peter: Can I take that further?

Edvin grunts.

Peter: Without the ability to think about your situation—without insight—you can't really see that you are unfree, and you can't decide to change. It's like the words of a new language and the insights and perspectives that these words bring. You can't change without that. You're stuck in your bubble. You can't do other than be angry and alienated—never really knowing why. You end up blaming yourself. It's like that junior doctor—we've met her—hasn't eaten for hours, hasn't slept, doesn't have the time to pee, running around the hospital like a chattering monkey with a list of jobs as long as her arm and no prospect of an end, and all the time old guys like us are holding over her this idea that she should be *kind*, or *compassionate*, or *wise*, and all *she* wants is to get home to feed her child. So the junior doc's thinking "I'm the only lousy doctor in the shop." That doctor has no capacity to critique. Only to suffer.

Edvin: I am not sure it's language she needs. It's courage. Power. Confidence.

Peter: And pain. But she needs the words to channel that.

Edvin: OK, you're right. The alternative is that dark suspicion—lying there like a stone in the mind. *I'm just not good enough.*

Peter: The only explanation she has.

Edvin and Peter, in their separate heads, have the same memory-image from the conference this spring. A circle of doctors, listening to a younger woman colleague, who is in tears—brave tears here—an honest confession is being made. They are sitting in a glass-walled room overlooking a bay. There is a calm blue sea, a gentle breeze. The makings of coffee on the floor around them at their feet. Later they will have a break. But now they are at work. She looks at her feet, teardrops coursing her cheeks. "That was the moment," she says, "that was the moment when I realized that I just wasn't good enough."

Part 2: The Barrel

Below the summit cone there is a plateau. A broader, flatter, rocky place, with a steep descent to the valleys on its flanks. It's distinctly colder now. The wind is getting up, and the hill fog funnels up around them, sudden, like smoke, blinding the walkers to their surroundings. Edvin and Peter shiver a little. They both know what it is to be lost in the hills, how that feels.

Peter thinks, as he does, from time to time, of the heart disease that killed most of the last few generations of his family. This half-suppressed thought: That for the last decade or so, he has been waiting for it. Waiting for it to begin. He takes a deep breath, clasps his fist to his chest, strides forth up the ascent. Thinks, no pain there! Not yet.

It can be hard on a mountain not to have thoughts of death. Perhaps it is the risk, the risk that is everywhere. Perhaps it is the abrupt fluctuations in the weather—one moment warm, the next, stormy and threatening. Perhaps it is the changed landscape, austere now, there is little that grows, no birds but the mountain ravens with their rattling, deep-throated calls.

Time perhaps to entertain BIG IDEAS.

Peter: We need to talk about the challenges involved. Something about choices of themes—how do you badge what the thing is about? Also, stuff about leadership—how does the power get distributed? Let's start with the theme of the conference. Is it necessary that there even *be* a theme? And if there must be, who chooses it? The problem's right there, right at the beginning. How to avoid creating oppressive forms of leadership? How does that work?

I have done this many times before, thinks Edvin, and Peter hasn't. How can I explain, in words that will make sense, how the thing just . . . emerges? How to explain the steps of a process that can seem, in the moment when it succeeds, like there is no hand behind it, like it's just a series of coincidences? This, it seems, is part of the task.

Edvin: My experience is that *having* a choice of theme matters—but the specific choice, less so. You can choose any topic from a big barrel of highly relevant themes—things about which we are truly curious, questions about life, and medicine, and what is right and wrong, and how we can know, and how we can make decisions when we cannot know. The function of the theme is not to offer a problem that we can solve at the conference. It is to create a shared feeling of being on a quest for understanding that is both professionally relevant and personally adventurous.

Peter: This "barrel of ideas?"

Edvin: They have certain things in common. They are problems of a philosophical kind that are common to all of us.

Peter: But become *salient* in medicine.

Edvin: Where they *fizz*. With uncertainty and relevance.

Peter: They are immanent in medicine but rarely taught to medical students.

221

Edvin: That may be because they are not easily grasped by any analytical tools. Hard to research. Impossible to measure. Easier to discuss. Questions like:

What is empathy?

Peter: What is personhood?

Edvin: What is autonomy? And then: What is care, and why should we care?

Peter: What is dignity?

Edvin: What is care, what is it to be good?

Peter: Hah! Old favourites.

Edvin: So many themes in the barrel, so much that can be used to create processes of thinking together. They are points of entry to the rich landscapes of "The Right Stuff of Medicine," useful ideas floating on the periphery of medical education, laden with doubt and indeterminacy.

Peter: Making life . . . complicated.

Edvin: And richer. Better. Truer. And not just for doctors. Here's another thought about how to navigate when you wish to create conditions for fertile thinking in a group of highly experienced people. It's easier to identify what you mustn't do than create rules for the things you must.

Peter: So the *process* becomes the significant issue, rather than the theme.

Edvin: Yes, as we just talked about, you need to create trust, so you must not belittle people—there is a lot to say about that. But the choice of intellectual theme is *also critical*. It can't just be bland. It has to invite people in. It can't be babble. Not all words or themes have the right kind of quality. It needs to provoke interest, without prescribing content.

Peter: We've talked about the choice of themes. What about the choice of people? How does that happen?

Part 3: The Why

Now we are standing on the summit. It is always cold up here. The winds never stop. There is no view to speak of—everything is lost in shifting fog. The ghosts of other walkers rear up out of the mist and then are gone.

Peter: Who are we doing this for?

Edvin: And why are we doing it?

Peter: Which surely are related questions.

Edvin: If we didn't start such a group, would one have generated spontaneously? And if so, by whom? How? I don't think it would. Medical norms are very powerful. They're persuasive. And unintentionally suppressive of other ways of thinking. And being.

Peter: So do we just invite along converts? People who are outsiders anyway? Or identify as "outsiders?" Those others who already experience dissatisfaction when occupying this medical role?

Edvin: If you divulge your own struggles of feeling sometimes like a medical outsider, others will hear you, and come to you. Like KE, super competent doctor, in some ways traditional in his attitudes, yet still riven with dissatisfaction.

Peter: So we attract people just like us! What fun (*not . . .*).

Edvin: That's the obvious risk. We need diversity. Age, experience, background, culture. Different kinds of people, with different eyes on the world of medicine. We had some, but nowhere near enough. It's a pervasive problem.

Peter: But at the same time, you need a vanguard of people who already speak and understand the language, who have the right kind of cognitive vocabulary. It sounds a bit old school communist—a revolutionary vanguard . . . but it's hard to get away from. The change doesn't happen just by itself. It needs a push. People who are already a little bit outside. We know who they are. But you never answered the question.

Edvin: ??

Peter: Why are *you* doing this?

Edvin: Because I need to understand things better. And I guess I'm hungry for the company of people who share that need. It's not just an intellectual thing: It feels much too risky and fragile for that. It's deeper than that. If it wasn't, it wouldn't be worth the pain. It's as if engaging in this kind of creative activity is something that a particular kind of person, to flourish, can't avoid doing.

Peter: And this has something to do with how you choose delegates.

Says Peter, who has the glimmering of an understanding.

Smart people, who want to lean into their own ignorance to *know* it. People who are *hungry* for what they don't know. But . . . if you're *really* starting from ignorance . . . you can't even begin to know your end point.

So how then do you know you're en route?

Edvin: Because it's signposted. You know the route because it gives you recognizable emotions. It's full of interest, it has resonance (Rosa, 2018). Joy, as we talked about. Playfulness, and a sense of relevance, the rewarding feeling that *this* is a deeper aspect of the theme we are exploring.

Peter: You might be able to give some kind of advance formulation dictating the purpose of a seminar, but it's the doing of it that tells you whether you're on track. The praxis. The satisfaction, the fun: It's the litmus paper. Yes, joy matters. It's in our nature: We're programmed to like that which is deeply significant. It makes our survival more likely.

Edvin: We need to hang on to that. Let joy be the compass: Consider satisfaction, its importance, in the evolutionary sense. Being good at something brings pleasure. If your thing—what it is you're doing, brings you joy—then you're on a good journey. But that presupposes jeopardy. Self-criticism. Risk. It's deeper than simple hedonistic pleasure.

Peter: But how do you tell the difference? Between OK pleasure, and the kind that isn't OK?

Edvin: Yeah, how can joy serve as a compass? It's easy to think of pleasures that aren't related to this "being on the right track" of some . . . virtuous, philosophical quest—hah! So how do we know that THIS joy is the right kind—the reward for virtue, for audacity, and growth? Maybe "virtue" is the helpful idea here. So: I am only truly, persistently, uncomplicatedly joyful if I behave in such a way that others trust me and I have a clean conscience. So, if I were wasting givers' funding and participants' time and energy, I couldn't enjoy all that good weather, singing, and companionship. Guilt and lying sucks life out of things. Kills the hope, the joy. And I guess our choice of theme, as long as it's from our "barrel of ideas," serves its purpose here. It provides a rule by which we can judge what we do—we steer by that overarching purpose of the seminar to explore ways of supporting human change and growth. I like the compass metaphor: My joy vanishes if what we do seems trite or banal, if it lacks risk or difficulty, or direction, or ambition. It's only if all of those conditions are met—honestly working on the theme; honestly daring to be in touch with ignorance, fallibility, vulnerability, and unexpected strengths and insights; honestly believing that people are becoming healthier versions of themselves—that I, as a leader, will experience genuine joy.

Peter: When we were in Roshven, It wasn't just pure, libidinous, fun. It connected to something deep, something that seemed categorically good. We were trying to learn to be better healers. Better people. Sure, we had a great time, but, arguably, that didn't detract from anyone, quite the opposite, it motivated everyone for honest, sometimes painful, thinking and sharing of stories and doubts. So it was more than just a holiday. Ninety-five per cent of the time, our hedonism connected to this deep, more profound sense of purpose. A Categorically Good Thing.

Or is this all just self-justifying, self-serving? And how would you know?

A moment's doubt creeps in.

Edvin: Peter, you make me think that what we are talking about now, and identify as joy, are ways of being together, as persons and professionals, that create optimism.

We reach the top of the hill, and then we push on—further into the cold. We descend a broad ridge, rocks, mud, some jeopardy as the ground shears away on both sides to cliffs. We've done the easy cone of Bein Vorlich. Now we approach the altogether more austere, rocky crag of Stuc á Chroin. It takes its shape, emerging from the cloud.

Peter: Optimism? What grounds can there ever be for optimism?

Edvin: Optimism is grounded in reason.

It's the evolutionary significance of joy. It is what carries you forward. Part of the nature of people is to engage in philosophy and speculation. Dialectical oppositions are hard-wired into our intellect—if you are aware, and rational, then you cannot help but engage in speculation. These processes are, by their nature, processes of constructive optimism. Any activity of making, of finding, building, changing, acting on the world— even simply of being—are, in their nature, optimistic. Doing. As opposed to its opposite.

Peter: Its opposite?

Edvin: Not doing. That loss of creativity. The loss of forward motion. That's a formulation for suffering. Optimism is the opposite to suffering.

Peter: A categorical formulation. A dyad of optimism versus suffering. Kindness and optimism, the core for everything that is good.

As if from nowhere a voice echoes through the suddenly still air.

An old woman.

It's lovely to hear two young men chatting away like that! Kindness! Optimism!

An old woman, half-hidden behind a rock, pokes out her head.

She leans back, reaches behind herself, deep into a recess or crack in the rock behind her. She pulls out a banana. Winks, conspiratorial, peels it, takes a bite.

People don't talk enough. In my view. And especially not like that. About their emotions and stuff. About what they really think! Kindness! Optimism! You should talk to my husband. A miserable bugger! Never says a word. A woman would die of boredom in his company. Kindness? Optimism? Doesn't know what these words mean! Are you going up Stuc á Chroin?

She nods at the crag—the jumble of rock, rising steeply in front of us, out of the mist. We grunt. We are.

Take care. It's longer, harder than you might think. And don't follow the path. It's deceptive—it turns to nothing. You want to scramble up the rocks to the left. It's steeper—a bit gnarly—a little fearsome—but it's safer in the end, and far more enjoyable.

We thank her and go on. Behind us, she rises stiffly to her feet. She throws down her banana skin. It is swallowed by the rock. She leans on her stick, says "Oof," and walks on, wobbling a little as she finds her feet.

We leave her behind in the fog. We begin our ascent. We avoid the path.

Edvin: That links back to my earlier—enormous—claim. That engaging in this makes you better at everything that you do.

Peter: Yes, a kind of focused optimism, that is Our Thing. It gives us tools to critique the system that forms us. You can only fight against despair if you have the tools. That's what I meant when I was talking about "language." The right language, making you better at everything that you do.

Edvin: Perhaps by conferring some immunity to self-hatred. Immunity to burnout.

| *Peter:* | Vaccine development. There's a future in *that!* To burnout. Someone should surely pay us! |

The two friends fall silent now. They are on steep, unstable rock. They must use hands and feet to ascend, there are moments where a fall would have consequences. They see the path the old woman indicated they avoid, how welcoming it looks at first, and then how narrow it becomes, before it disappears. They pull themselves to the top, drink tea from carved wooden cups, nibble chocolate, begin their slow descent.

Part 4: Embodying Wisdom

Now we are on miserable terrain. Endless mud, paths snaking off in all directions through the bog and heather. All walks have their tiresome sections. We fire off quick thoughts about the form and organization of our seminar. Logistics! Preparation! Program! Sequencing events! Activate participants at every opportunity!

The weather has cleared, there is a view across the loch, to the massif of blue hills opposite, Beinn Lawers, an Stac, the Ptarmigan Ridge, and all the ranges to the north of that.

| *Edvin:* | It would not have succeeded unless everyone took part, despite disparity of experience and expertise. There were no exceptions in the group. No free-riders. Nowhere to hide. Everyone had to help carry it. All participants were warned and knew they would have to be active. The young and less experienced doctors knew tons from personal experience that the seniors can learn from, and vice versa. Daring to think aloud, and being listened to, participants were validated and united. |

| *Peter:* | Then the choice of location, obviously. Somewhere special. Four days, the 24-hour presence of people. You need that, that affirmation. Immersion. It needs to be immersive. |

| *Edvin:* | Yes, because the group relationships, to be affected by the ways others act, the way they meet you and talk to you, is the most powerful source of change. There was a plan, there |

was a lot of structure. But the participants were uncertain what was expected of them when they arrived. After about 24 hours of noticing that there are reasonable and flexible plans and that slips are acknowledged and corrected, people start to have trust and to accommodate the structure, the rhythms, the timing. The group creates its own discipline. The "leader" role seems to fade away. The precise time keeping, the planned activities that involve everyone, having sufficient space for rest and reflection—these remain essential—but it's the person who is talking, or the group that is presenting, who becomes the real source of authority. The leaders ideally melt into the background, can learn together with everyone and be stewards of the stuff that emerges when people are at their best, together. The right stuff, sort of.

Peter: I remember the preparations. There was a real preoccupation with logistics. All those meetings when we sat on the floor with great sheets of paper and coloured pens, planning, planning. And the emails to the group in the months before. Each sentence designed to get that balance between raising expectation, a little trepidation, yet maintaining a sense of safety. That sense of being invited in. To be unconditionally part of the group, and yet.

Edvin: We did our best to create high expectations. Both ways. But it was safe, wasn't it?

Peter: Safe? Not that safe. What about the "Being" sessions?

Interior: Peter's head.

We were asked, each of us, to bring an artefact—something that we might use to present ourselves, to tell our stories (see Chapters 10 *and* 11*).*

I had brought with me a little black notebook. My dad had written in it a week or two before he died. He knew he was getting to his end. He wrote this quote:

"Nature I have loved, and after nature, art. I have warmed my hands before the fire of life, and now I am ready to depart."

He was telling me—instructing me, in the clearest possible way—that he was dying and how he wanted to do it. What a charge! What a gift! He was teaching me, in turn, how to die.

And I told you guys about it. I remember, I choked up. You guys, in a horseshoe, listening. And you were quiet afterwards, because you had recognized something, and understood. It felt risky—it felt riskier than anything that I had done since . . . I don't know . . . since I was a child. Yet it was also safe.

He sniffs hard on the cooling air.

Edvin: Those "being sessions . . ."

For a bit, they tramp across a moor, picking steps between those deep black peat stanks, minds focused, lost in recollection.

Peter: Do you remember, lying on our backs on the floor, whilst Caroline beat a huge oriental gong. How you could feel it, vibrating through your bones!

Edvin: Do you remember the singing games—"John's got a pingpong pingpong head"? How everyone, in the end, joined in, singing, together!

Peter: All that barefoot shouting at the sea. All the profanities, all that yelling at the poor old fish.

Edvin: The focused silence. That sense of all being together, all committed, all participating.

Peter: The sharing of confidences. A lot of honesty.

We sat under an old, thick, twisted rowan tree and admired its indecent fruit. It's late September. It's still warm. The colour scheme is full of red, shades of yellow, browns, and some gold. As the conversation progresses, the sun begins to set, shadows grow long, the colours grow richer. It's the loveliest time of year. A warm breeze is coming from the west.

We are back down now. And, of course, the weather has cleared. The sun is fully out, we are back, on flat, easy ground.

Peter: I still have my pill box.

At the end of each of these strange, disparate experiences we had shared out to each a little, coloured bead of natural stone, a marble. We put it in a pill box, as if it were a drug, a prescription that we might take and use to ease our own suffering—ease our suffering with a dose of memory—of sun-drenched electric days by the sea, when the sky was blue and the rain held off for four days straight, when we lay on our backs whilst Caroline beat her gong, or we yelled at the sea, or we sang in wavering harmony whilst Victoria, the choir mistress's daughter, kept us, more or less, together.

Peter: I keep it on a shelf in my consulting room. I take it down from time to time and rattle it, or hold the coloured beads between my fingers, and remember.

All that planning we did! Yet how little of it we used!

Edvin: The planning was essential. The actual plans less important.

★   ★   ★

The rest, more or less, was rambling.

We sat a while longer under our rowan tree. Admiring its orange berries, the way the light and shadow flickered through the fingers of its leaves.

Edvin told a story. About some chestnuts he had found and picked up in a park in Rouen, France, where he had lived a while, a lonely year, as a schoolboy. He'd picked them up because, although adolescent, at heart he was a bairn still and still loved his conkers, their shimmer and varnish, and he longed for childhood, and he missed his mother and his home.

And how, when at last he had got home, he had carelessly thrown them away in the garden of his mother's cabin by the fjord, just forgot about them.

And how, years later, one autumn, middle-aged now—let's be frank, not so far off old—he had found an alien chestnut leaf—so out of place!—browning on the sand at the water's edge, of what is now his cabin, and, tracing these leaves back up a muddy slope, had found in the remnants of his mother's garden a grove of forgotten saplings, growing: Chestnuts! From Rouen.

Healthy, thriving, unintended.

References

Kahneman, D. (2011). *Thinking, fast and slow* (1st ed.). Farrar, Straus and Giroux.

Rosa, H. (2018). The idea of resonance as a sociological concept. *Global Dialogue, 8*(2), 41–44.

Rudebeck, C. E. (2001). Grasping the existential anatomy: The role of bodily empathy in clinical communication. In *Handbook of phenomenology and medicine* (pp. 297–316). Springer.

Shapiro, J. (2011). Perspective: Does medical education promote professional alexithymia? A call for attending to the emotions of patients and self in medical training. *Academic Medicine, 86*(3), 326–332. https://doi.org/10.1097/ACM.0b013e3182088833

18

End

Peter Dorward

A year or so after the last time we met—this little group of ours, this precious band of friends—I had rather a bad time of it. Nothing much, but enough to notice. Something not quite right. My bad time lasted for about a month. There were three causes, I think, insofar as one can ever really know the proper causes of such passing darknesses.

The first event, the one that set the tone, the key signature for this short bad time, makes most sense to everyone, and so is the easiest to describe.

My mother-in-law died. But she was a hundred years old! And *so* ready to die. Death is only a problem, a philosopher friend of mine once said, when she visits too early, or too late. It was intolerable to my mother in law that she was old—that this, her welcome end, came so delayed. Despite the love and care that surrounded her, she felt the indignity of her situation keenly.

The funeral was on a hot day. Beforehand, a small group of us sat under a tree in a garden and counted the red kites that were wheeling like dragons in the thermals above the crematorium chimneys. After, family and friends ate and drank in the yard of a pub near Oxford and talked and told stories, and we enveloped ourselves in the affection that we all had had for this . . . extraordinary person. Sadness will often seed itself in this kind of warm, nourishing soil. I left early. I had to be at work the next morning. I had a long journey.

When I arrived at work the next morning, I discovered that a patient of mine had died. I was tired—the trains were delayed, as they always are, and

DOI: 10.1201/9781003593294-18

I had got in very late. I *thought* I was fine though. But this person's death was the second proximate cause of my unhappiness.

The death was expected. A short illness.

He had presented to me just seven weeks earlier, with non-specific abdominal pain. I ran a bunch of tests, they were all normal. When he came back to see me a week after, for the results, his pain was already gone. But he wanted to see me anyway, he said—he wanted to thank me. Not for this, our most recent transaction, but for our previous contact, five or so years previously, when he had had a personal crisis—something to do with his work and his family. He wanted to thank me for *listening* to him. For the uncritical quality of this listening, he said, for the fact that I hadn't given him advice or told him what to do.

"So," he said, shaking my hand, "I wanted to thank you, and give you this."

A card, with a book token. It was a little awkward, perhaps, but moving, and I was intensely flattered.

He was almost exactly my age, and we had a great overlap of interests. We read the same books and talked about them. In other circumstances, we might have been friends; we almost were.

He called me back, a week or so later. I saw his name on my list, an emergency, I had that familiar, discreditable doctor's reflex—*have I missed something?*—but I hadn't. He was in a state. It wasn't the previous pain back, he thought, it was something else—some global distress, some not-rightness, that evaded him, something had stooped and *seized* him and wouldn't let him go. It was beyond him to describe it—and he never would—he never quite found the words to name what ailed him.

I saw him early the next morning. I think that he had lost weight since our last meeting. He looked like a fugitive—wide frightened eyes, hunched, on the run, his shadow following, half a step behind.

"And now I have this!" he said pointing and grimacing at his neck. Since earlier that morning, he had developed a large, pulsatile mass arising just above his left clavicle.

We doctors get to know death, at least we think we do. Her various avatars. This is our business, to know her.

Death, as an efficient, fine-bladed pair of scissors. *Snip.*

Death as a capacious, comforting shroud that gathers and holds us at our ends.

The harvester.

The force that drops the sparrow from the tree.

The incompetent bike mechanic that didn't quite get to tighten the nut right.

But today, it's her ravenous side: The one she rarely shows, but can, at any time:

> Ragged, grimy, shit-smeared, grave-stained, shrieking *You! You! You!*, dressed in thin cotton shift printed with rose-buds, gripped between her bony knees a half-dead mule which she thrashes with a switch of nettle hemp; in her right hand she waves this dripping bread-knife and she is coming for us, one of us, faster than we can hope to get away, and so we just stand there, transfixed, powerless as she comes. *You! You! You!*

We were always one step behind, it seemed. One step behind his final diagnosis; the treatments for this diagnosis, which were few; his symptoms, which were many, various, and hard to pin down; his fear, which held him fast, almost to his end.

There is a form that needs to be signed when death happens, affixed to the patient's paper records. I think *I'm fine,* as I write my initials in the box, though probably I'm not, quite.

But it was the third event that really did it for me. So trivial. It was nothing really.

It was nothing!

Right at the bottom of my list of *stuff to do* lurked a request for a prescription marked *urgent,* for some drug or other that was the *wrong* drug—it's always the wrong drug, and it's never, by definition, urgent. It only becomes urgent because he's angry. An angry man. Codeine. Zopiclone. Anusol. Enough to make a man mad.

I had bumped the request that morning, and I had bumped it again that afternoon, not knowing that someone else had bumped it the previous evening.

I had other stuff to do. A young woman is in the waiting room, who may, or may not, be cutting, and may or may not, seriously hurt herself. There are two calls waiting for feverish children, and there is a fact to check—a thing I had told a patient an hour or so ago as if it were God's own truth, of which I am now far less certain, and I know I need to fix that. *That's* urgent.

Every day, sorting through these fragile parcels, each one precious to its sender, some heavy, some light, some unmarked.

And now the phone rings and my receptionist tells me that the angry man has turned up in person, and sure enough, now that I am aware, I can hear raised voices.

What can I do? Don't be such an arse. Just give him his prescription! For the *wrong* drug.

Or ask the receptionist to ask this angry, shouty man to just go away. He'll tear into her. He's known for it. It's what he does. And she's off to Prague this weekend with her boyfriend, she's *really* looking forward to it, she's been telling everyone about it.

So squander what time and compassion you have on the angry man, see him, deal with this tiny matter yourself.

Which I say I'll do. The receptionist is really grateful. "I'll just ask him to sit down and wait."

The angry man stands up as soon as I appear, jabbing his forefinger at his watch.

A thin young woman dressed in black—my waiting patient—glances up. She flinches a little at the force of him as he passes, thinking, no doubt, how much more important than she he must be, that she must wait, still, a little longer. But *she* won't complain.

Angry Jack Savage, as he is unironically named, has no such scruples, jumping right in before he is halfway down the corridor.

"It's an absolute disgrace! How you think you can treat people!"

He's probably right—thinks that almost smothered, yet still rational part of me.

He sits down, carefully places on the table between us an iPhone, screen down, looks pointedly at it for a moment, says, "I want an explanation, and I want it now. Why you think it's OK to leave a sick person waiting for his medication, for more than a day?"

I look at his iPhone. I look at him, and I think, probably rightly, *the whole world can listen in.* And then I think, also rightly, *and today, today I just can't be arsed with this.*

I put the shutters down on what kindness I might have had left. Compassion is my most precious, my only, resource.

I tell him that in this little slot of time we have, you and I, I can try to manage your medical problem, but not your anger. *I can't do both.* I have no time to manage your anger—but he is just outraged by this, and a part of me knew he would be.

"… are you trying to tell me that …?"

"I'm not *trying* to tell you anything," I say, as I stand, to open the door, "I'm *telling* you that I have no time to deal with your anger."

All my fancy theories about *suffering.* All that stuff about *listening. Compassion. Wisdom.* All out the window in a flash.

You see, I'm not *trying* here to tell a story about how this doctor was the smartest, or wisest, or bravest person in the room. We rarely are, and I'm a little tired of these kinds of stories. I'm trying to tell a story about how he was the stupidest. The vainest. The one more blinded by power and passion. That feels truer. Vainglory. I think that that's a story worth telling, today, at least.

"Then I'm going to have it out with that girly at the desk. This is a joke."

"No you're not," I say. "You're leaving."

"So are you telling me now who I can and can't speak with?"

"Yes."

Men who have done time generally know when to stop. The ones that don't are still doing time.

Many of my Rules for Life are unreliable. Some are frankly dangerous. This being one of them.

No sooner is Jack Savage gone then there is a knock at my door. It's my trainee. Ruth. She says, "Are you alright? I heard raised voices." She is appalled to see tears rising, filling up my eyes. Old men don't cry. That's another one of my Rules for Life.

It wasn't Jack Savage who undid me. He, at the end of the day, was blameless in this. It was the kindness of my colleague.

★   ★   ★

We met as a group twice—the first for a few days in Rosendal. Spring, in a farmhouse on the shore of the great Hardangerfjord in the south-west of Norway. The second in Rósvein, a tiny fjord, on the north-west coast of Scotland. We were graced by sun, warm weather, and blue seas both times.

We tasked ourselves with these topics that we had chosen, taken from this great barrel of other, related topics, and we found ourselves with many more. We laughed a lot, we made music, we ate, drank, argued, fought a bit.

We formalized accounts of our meetings, refined them, edited them down, made them into a book.

This is that book.

The experience of the magic and accumulated wisdom of these seminars has made me better, in every way. As a doctor, as a person.

I can give no evidence to stand this claim up, other than knowing it, with certainty, to be true. Which, of course, is no kind of evidence at all.

★   ★   ★

"So, remind me. What is the point of all of this?"

It's my trainee's last tutorial. The one whose kindness so undid me.

We're standing at the top of a low hill looking east, out to sea. It's the dead of winter. Clear blue sky, cold as cold can be, the sun barely rising in the south.

"I don't know. I can't really remember."

So often it's the simplest questions that floor me.

"You tell me."

That's the teacher's last, often only, resort.

"I think," she says to me, and I am quiet, because usually what she says makes a lot of sense, "I *think* it's about learning how to be kind. I mean the right *kind* of kind. In a world that can seem structurally, intentionally bereft of that skill. And learning how to *keep* doing it. Over and over, until the end. I *think* that that is the point."

OK, I think. That works.

Index

For Product Safety Concerns and Information please contact our EU
representative GPSR@taylorandfrancis.com
Taylor & Francis Verlag GmbH, Kaufingerstraße 24, 80331 München, Germany

* 9 7 8 1 0 3 2 9 7 3 3 3 3 *